Joanne Reynolds has offered a pri
by hard circumstance—the serious
travel this most challenging road. Writing with a deft confidence as a trustworthy and patient guide, she blends her personal experience along with the insights she has gleaned from other authorities in the field. Although Reynolds writes as a person of faith, the respectful tone of this book will endear it to anyone willing to learn important and heartfelt lessons common to all who navigate this journey with and for another. People of faith may recognize *Search for Light* to be not merely informative and helpful but even redemptive. Quite an accomplishment for a smallish book.

—Pastor Chip Fisher

I devoured the first eight chapters.

—Rev. Judee Archer Green

How wonderful! Your writing is like having a conversation with a dear and knowing friend. It's been comforting to me to read your explanations of the process and procedures. Being informed helps so much in dealing with our anxiety. Your book is full of words of wisdom and so helpful in encouraging the patient and caregiver.

—Delrena Sides

I thought I knew about caregiving; after all, I'm a pastor. That is, until my ninety-three-year-old mother-in-law moved in with us. I thank God for your book! I found out how much I had to learn.

—Rev. Wilma Houston White

I've had participants from your workshop contacting me about the book. They all appreciate the valuable information.

—Karin Stewart

There is so much information Joanne gives about everything that can happen to people going through all this. She has *so* many hands-on stories of all the experiences that are very helpful. Her details really enlighten as to what truly *does* happen.

—Peggy Moore

This little gem, written from a caregiver's perspective, is a helpful roadmap for those caring for loved ones with a life-threatening illness. It is a must-read for all who are new to the caregiver's role.

—Dorothy Siddall, MD, FAAFP Professor of Family Medicine

This book is a must-read for anyone caring for a loved one. I only wish this book was available when I had to arrange care for my mother and then my mother-in-law through long, drawn-out terminal afflictions. The lessons on how to be sure to take care of yourself first so you have the strength to carry on for your family is invaluable. The knowledge that some residual effects can continue to devastate the caregiver long after the actual event comes to closure was especially enlightening to me. I am actively pursuing an end to my own personal residual effects using Joanne's edifying labor of love and sharing.

—Carolyn Gaylord

Through telling the poignant stories of her own experiences, Joanne Reynolds develops a series of concrete suggestions to help caregivers realize the gift they have been given as well as the amazing gift they can give to people they love.

—John F. Llewellyn
Author of *Saying Goodbye Your Way*

search *for* LIGHT

search *for*
LIGHT

Ten Crucial
Lessons for
Caregivers

Joanne Reynolds

TATE PUBLISHING *& Enterprises*

Published by Tate Publishing & Enterprises, LLC
127 E. Trade Center Terrace | Mustang, Oklahoma 73064 USA
1.888.361.9473 | www.tatepublishing.com

Tate Publishing is committed to excellence in the publishing industry. The company reflects the philosophy established by the founders, based on Psalm 68:11,
"The Lord gave the word and great was the company of those who published it."

Book design copyright © 2009 by Tate Publishing, LLC. All rights reserved.
Cover design by Lance Waldrop
Interior design by Stefanie Rooney

Published in the United States of America

ISBN: 978-1-60799-968-3
1. Health & Fitness, General 2. Family & Relationships, Eldercare
09.10.01

DEDICATION

To MaryKay. I miss you, sis.

ACKNOWLEDGMENTS

The effort to bring this book to reality has involved many people. I would like to acknowledge and give thanks to:

Cheryl Dumler and Cynthia Hollern, who were its inspiration; the members of my sharing group, who offered valuable emotional and spiritual support throughout this long learning process; Art Vinsel, a good friend and talented writer, who is a most capable copy editor; Heather Moreno, whose own book inspired me to revisit this one and who brought her eagle eye to the hunt for typos; Carol and John Llewellyn, dear relations who are such gentle critics; Peggy Moore, who so thoughtfully and thoroughly reviewed the final manuscript; Linda Short, a fearless friend who was willing to brave the hunt for a publisher when I tired of rejection letters, and Wyndi Bradley, whose life is so filled with grace that she could see possibilities I could not even imagine.

In addition, I owe a great debt of thanks for the competence and caring of Jaime McNutt Bode, my excellent editor, and all of the wonderful people on the staff of Tate Publishing.

Most of all, I want to acknowledge all of the family, friends and newly-met caregivers who have brought me so many blessings in caregiving. You are in my heart, always.

PREFACE

April 26, 1998

Today, after church, I was telling Carol about MaryKay's recurrence of cancer. Carol is a sympathetic personality by nature, but since her mom died of cancer, it seemed natural to go ahead and spill out all of my fears and frustrations— not knowing what to do, how to help MK, whether to put my upcoming retirement on hold, and on and on. I'm so glad I picked her to vent with. When I finally sputtered to a stop, she patted my arm gently. "Don't worry about doing anything in particular," she said. "Just hold her hand."

This book is written for those of you who find yourselves in similar circumstances, facing serious illness or injury, or perhaps even terminal diagnosis of a loved one—a family member or dear friend. While much of what I want to share with you can also apply to the ill or injured person and the process they are undergoing, for the most part, this book is intended for—and dedicated to—the family and friends who are rallying behind their loved one, trying to find answers to the question, *What are we going to do?*

The caregiving that I'm talking about here includes *all*

of the things you will be doing for your loved one, in addition to the medical treatment and skilled nursing that he or she is receiving. Whether you have taken on the enormous job of being the live-in, full-time caregiver or whether you are someone who comes by regularly to spend time with the ill or injured person, my thoughts, ideas, and experiences are addressed directly to you. This book is for family and friends who are not medical professionals. It is written for all of you who are feeling as helpless as the patient but who want *to do* something.

In writing this book, I held in my mind the picture of an adult—anyone from twenty-something to eighty-something—whose loved one is ill or injured. You are the people who live with the patient or share deep bonds of friendship and family. I wrote this for those of you who will provide care at home after the hospital stay is over and who will prepare the meals, drive the patient to appointments, pick up medications and equipment, support the therapy or exercise regimen, or simply visit and listen to your loved one.

My frame of reference for *caregiver* includes all those who shift their schedules to make themselves available on a regular basis to a loved one who is ill or injured. Caregivers range from the spouses and life partners who share a home with the patient to the family and friends who make themselves available to help in some way on a regular basis.

All of you who are taking on this new responsibility have a special place in my heart. I know how difficult the work is that you've taken on, and I urge you to take care of yourself while you're caring for the ill person. Your well-being is a vitally important part of what you have to offer your loved one.

My Story

Most of the information I offer here I have come by through experience. More than thirty years ago I helped care for my mother, Kay Shaw, while she fought her cancer, and I was present as she died. I also helped to care for my grandmother, Louisa Shaw, who slowly succumbed to the ravages of Parkinson's disease. Not long after that, my beloved mother-in-law, Annette Reynolds, began her final journey through her fight with cancer. Most importantly, from 1998 until 1999, I cared for and supported my only sister, MaryKay Crookall, as she dealt with her cancer. Once again, as with our mother, I was able to be at her side and share the moment when she left this physical life.

Certainly not all of the family encounters with serious illness have been fatal. My sister-in-law, Rosemarie, has had her own struggles with cancer and is now enjoying a prolonged period of remission. My stepbrother, Tom, was diagnosed with multiple sclerosis in 2001 and at present is leading an active life.

The inspiration for this book came out of the serious, but short-term, illness of two close, lifelong friends. When Cindy and Cheryl were both diagnosed with breast cancer, just preceding and following my sister's death, I was moved to write about what I have learned specifically from her illness and from my part in caring for her. At the same time, I have come to realize that *all* the experiences of being with and caring for family or friends with serious illnesses or life-threatening injury have added to my store of knowledge. My experience—hands-on, sometimes day-to-day—is a large part of what I have to offer here.

Sadly, the opportunities to practice these principles and ideas do not end. My father, Don Shaw, started his battle in 1991 with testicular cancer. He developed a secondary lymphoma in

1997 and a leukemia-like blood condition in 1999. In late 2002, Dad's condition began to deteriorate, with hospitalizations for antibiotic-resistant infections. With the assistance of his wife, Claudette, he fought his infections and dealt with his blood condition while he did what he could to maintain his work and personal life until he died in August 2003. What care I was privileged to give to Dad was profound in its own way, yet very different from the experiences I had with my sister and with other family members whose illnesses preceded his.

Then in 2004, my young cousin, William, died of kidney cancer. Two months before his death, William left his wife and three young sons at their home in the French Alps to come back to Southern California to undergo a *very* alternative therapy. He stayed for a time with my husband and me, and during that time, I realized I was still learning new lessons about what it means to be a caregiver. While my experiences with Dad and William were considerably different than with my sister, they have expanded my understanding of caregiving and are an important part of what I have to offer you.

Information from Experts

Beyond my own experiences, the lessons I offer here come from books written by and about patients and the people who cared for them, and from stories in the press. Look in your daily newspaper or in the magazines in the supermarket, and you will see these stories on a regular basis, accounts of people who are struggling with disease or injury and how they manage to cope—or not—because of the assistance of family and friends. If you are reading this book, then you are in a similar circumstance, and I recommend that you keep an eye out for the books and news stories that contain accounts of patients and their supporters. You may find them helpful to you in your process.

Over the past three years, I have continued to learn about caregiving by teaching classes and leading workshops. Every time I meet with a caregiver—or a group of them—I learn something new. The anecdotes I offer in this book come from my own experience, from the work of experts, and, recently, from the caregivers I've encountered from across the country. Whether they are caring for dementia patients, they are hospice volunteers, or they are preparing themselves for a future role as a caregiver, each individual has brought me continuing lessons in compassion in action, which is the true work of caregiving.

I want to emphasize that what I have to offer is anecdotal, stories about experiences, not data out of scientific studies. This book contains the widest range of information from my experiences or the anecdotes of others that I could find. Not all of what's offered here will apply to you and your loved one. This is meant to be something of a buffet of ideas and suggestions from which you can choose the things that are the most appealing or which you believe will be the most helpful, and leave the rest behind.

You'll notice that each chapter opens with a short entry from my journal. These are representative thoughts and feelings that I recorded beginning with my sister's initial diagnosis in June 1997 through June 2000. I have included them so you can see the range of emotions that I experienced in being a caregiver and so you will understand how normal your emotional ups and downs are.

Organization of This Book

This book is organized into two sections, beginning with a three-lesson section entitled "Understanding Basic Concepts."

These first lessons include a more detailed telling of the stories of members of my family and how my search for light in those times of personal darkness led to the discovery of blessings; a description of the five stages of emotional processing of traumatic events first explained in 1969 by Dr. Elisabeth Kubler-Ross, and my understanding of the connection of the body, mind, and spirit.

This underlying information of these first three lessons is important for you to have in order to have a clear understanding of both the principles and practices I offer in the second section, "Putting the Basics to Work." The seven lessons in this section contain some general information: the diagnosis, the medical team, the patient, the patient's team, being with the patient, emotional/psychological support, and self-care for caregivers. While the first part of each lesson is general in nature, each ends with a specific list of suggestions under the heading "What You Can Do." You will probably notice that the material in the body of these chapters is sometimes repeated as a bulleted item in the "What You Can Do" section. I thought it important to keep the information in an easily-found format rather than having you search for it through the body of each lesson. I hope you will forgive the occasional repetition of material that's listed with new ideas.

The book concludes with a summary chapter, "Life Is Messy." As much as I would like to have entitled it with a thought on the order of "Life Is Tidy and Happy Endings Abound," that has not been my experience. Still, as messy as life gets—and it can get very messy indeed—it continuously reveals opportunities for blessings in the midst of chaos and darkness. The challenge we all face in these circumstances is to search for the light of those blessings rather than surrender to the darkness.

Asking

Having been where you find yourself now, I know the importance of asking—asking questions, asking for help, asking for time off from your caregiving duties, asking for training to give care more confidently, or asking for additional treatment options for your patient. The list of what to ask for is endless, but it starts with asking questions to gather information about this new and unexpected phase of your life.

I strongly recommend that you make use of the Internet to find the non-profit organizations that support the illness or injury condition which affects your loved one. These organizations can be a great starting point to understanding what your loved one is going through physically and emotionally and can point you to additional sources of information, such as local support groups. A visit to your local library is also a good place to start your information gathering. There you can find a variety of books that will further expand your knowledge of your loved one's condition.

Making use of the wisdom of others, specifically people who have professional credentials as physicians, therapists, and counselors, is an absolutely necessary component of what I've written here and in what you are doing in caring for your loved one. The information of these experts is based on scientific research, a lifetime of professional expertise, or personal experiences and can be of great help in the work you're undertaking. I am not trained in medicine of any kind or in psychology, and this book is not intended to be used as a medical or psychological therapeutic resource. I am offering these insights and suggestions simply because they worked for me or for others that I know of, and I hope they can assist you to be more effective in helping someone you love.

I share this information with you with two seemingly contradictory understandings:

First, each person's process is unique, and my experiences with ill loved ones may differ from yours. A personality is formed over a lifetime in response to events both good and bad, and so the response to the illness itself, the treatment process, and the ultimate outcome are going to be different for each individual.

Rabbi Ben Kamin, in his excellent book *The Path of the Soul,* notes that under the stress of a serious illness, people become more of what they truly are. If they are at heart prone to laughter, then that is what they will do more of; if anger is their basic operating emotion, then anger is what will be exhibited during the medical crisis. Each of us is a unique creation, and so the response to the illness and the treatment will likewise be unique.

Yet, at the same time, much of what I have to say is universal. As different as each individual may be in their physical, emotional, intellectual, and spiritual response to their illness or injury, they, and the people who care for them, are going to share some experiences that are common to everyone. For instance, Dr. Kubler-Ross, in outlining the stages of response to pending death—anger, denial, bargaining, depression, and acceptance—detailed a process that is universal to humanity and which applies not just to the process of dying but also to the process of illness, whether or not the illness results in death. Her description of these phases also applies to the people who care for the patient.

Patient and caregiver alike, we all work through these stages in response to the effect of the illness and treatment. While we are each unique, our responses under this great stress have some universal qualities to them. That just means that it's possible to learn from another's experiences.

My Goal for You

My goal with this book is to help you search for God's light in this time of darkness for you and your loved one. I want to give you the tools you'll need to come to the understanding that I have reached—caregiving is a privilege because you move into a very private and personal place with your loved one, a place that can be deeply intimate for both of you. I want to achieve this goal by providing you with ideas and suggestions that work, the processes and practices that are beneficial to the patient and you.

In a few places, I've also included examples of shadow experiences, the things that in my experience don't work, that obscure the light, or just make the time of darkness more difficult to bear by fostering hopelessness, fear, and anger. In presenting some of this negative information, my hope is that you'll be able to prepare yourself to accept it for what it is if it comes into your life during this time.

The greatest lesson, the brightest blessing that I discovered and hope will guide you to finding yourself, is learning the importance of *being* rather than always *doing*. It's a lesson about truly being with your loved ones, of willingness to set aside your to-do list in order to be fully and completely present to them. It's learning to really hear what they want and need to say about their life experiences and, in doing so, coming to a deeper acceptance of whom each of you are and what your individual lives mean to one another.

Finally, and most importantly, the information I have to offer, specifically about emotional and spiritual well-being, is based not only on my personal experience but also on my personal beliefs as a follower of Christ.

I firmly believe in a loving, merciful God who is immediately available to us throughout our lives. This amazing God is just as present in dealing with the illness or injury as the medical personnel, family, and friends who have gathered around the ill person. When the patient and the caregiver invoke this holy presence in the process of care, I believe new opportunities for growth and wholeness for all of you come into being. The work you are undertaking can be far more than just the day-to-day support of the medical treatment. I believe healing is possible, apart from treatment or cure, when you invite this divine power into partnership in the process.

Now is the season to know that everything you do is sacred and to likewise know that you are never alone in the process, whatever its outcome.

God bless you.

Lord, high and holy, meek and lowly, Thou has brought me to the valley of vision, where I live in the depths but see Thee in the heights … Lord, in the daytime stars can be seen from the deepest wells, and the deeper the wells the brighter Thy stars shine; let me find Thy light in my darkness … Thy glory in my valley.

(Taken from *The Valley of Vision: A Collection of Puritan Prayers and Devotions*, Arthur Bennett, editor.)

UNDERSTANDING BASIC CONCEPTS

LESSON ONE:
FINDING THE LIGHT

June 8, 2000, Flagstaff, Arizona

Ané and I have been working hard getting her garden in. Being out in the sun and the dirt and the sheer physicality of the work—dragging boulders to the garden, finding interesting old farm stuff to use for planters—has put us in a good place to reflect on MaryKay. Lots of talk about what we learned, whether we can carry it with us, how MaryKay's spirit infuses those lessons—that sort of spiritual/philosophical talk that she and I love to share. Her take is that caring for people who are sick or hurting physically isn't about their pain and suffering, nor is it about our goodness in taking care of them. Instead, it's about how both the caregiver and patient can grow by visiting their own baggage and then getting past it. She believes it's about the opportunities to mend the wounds we cause and heal the ones we've received. To my mind, that makes caregiving nothing less than an opportunity for redemption.

Our lives, on every level imaginable, follow patterns of light and darkness. Daily, we experience the spinning of our globe around the sun, with its hours of daylight and hours of nighttime. We have times of success when we're in the limelight, and there are times when we feel in the dark, not quite working up to our capabilities or in sync with our surroundings. In the same way, the arc of our lives also passes through times when it feels as if all the light of the universe is flowing through us, when divine forces seem to be focused on bringing us only good. But these times inevitably are followed by darker times. It's an inescapable fact of human existence.

We will always come round to *bad* times, times when we are beset by trials, during which it seems we are surrounded by darkness. And it is a very real part of those dark days that we feel as if we are lost and there is no discernible way to get out of the nighttime experiences we're having.

Serious illness—cancer, stroke, and diseases of the immune system, heart, liver, kidneys, and central nervous system—and life-altering injury bring on those dark times. I know. I've been through the process, in varying degrees of intensity, with a dozen friends and family, including both my mother and father, my only sister, my mother-in-law, my grandmother, my sister-in-law, and one of my cousins. Each time, I experienced the feelings of helplessness and despair at the suffering of the person I love, and I felt as if I were living through an endless nighttime as the medical treatments and re-diagnoses and more treatments slowly ticked by, month after month. These are indeed dark times for the patients and those who love and care for them.

However, darkness has an important quality, which we sometimes forget when we're in the midst of it, be it a physical dark or a time of emotional darkness. At those times, it's difficult for us to realize that *only* when there is darkness is there the ability for us to see light. Shine a flashlight on a sunny day and what happens? Not much. But shine that same flashlight at night, and suddenly, you have a means of seeing where you're going. If it weren't for night, we would never see the stars and would not be able to appreciate the silver beauty of the moon, because those more subtle lights can only shine clearly in darkness.

The same principle applies to our emotional states. When we're plunged into dark times, we have an opportunity to find sources of light—blessings—that we've not seen before. That is the one shining lesson I have learned through my periods of personal trial when loved ones were suffering from illness or injury. There are blessings to be accepted by everyone involved in the process, regardless of its outcome. Whether patients recover, go into remission, learn new lifestyles to accommodate a disability, or succumb to the illness or injury, I firmly believe they—and the caregivers who are close to them—have an unprecedented opportunity in the process to find new ways of being, to heal old wounds that restrain them from being most fully alive, and to discover the constant presence and love of God in their lives. Often, these kinds of blessings can only begin to come to light in darkness, in the face of injury, disease, and death.

While it is true that this great opportunity lies within the darkness of the illness or injury, not everyone will recognize it or seize it. Each individual is a distillation of genetics, family history, and personal experience, and so their reactions will be based on their physical, emotional, and spiritual makeup. What was true for my mother's process was not always true for my sister's. My grandmother's response to her disease differed in some important ways from my father's reaction to his disease. Sometimes we found the light together; sometimes they each did it on their own. And there were cases where there was little discovery of blessing, even though the potential for these healing discoveries was always present.

The opportunities to find this deeper meaning, these profound understandings, are not the only blessings to be found in these circumstances. When those of us who are closest to the patient allow ourselves to become attentive to the threat to life that the patient is faced with, we have an opportunity to change the way in which we view the precious gifts conferred on each of us each day by life. That can happen because the illness or injury forces us to slow down, drop our schedule-dominated lives, and take a new approach to discovering the small pleasures that life has to give. These *little blessings* are available to patient and caregiver alike and can arise out of giving and receiving small acts of kindness.

Life presents opportunities for moments of light brought out by beauty, love, and joy. Sometimes we need to be forced to slow ourselves down enough to capture those moments by appreciating the beauty of a blooming flower or sharing an everyday experience with a loved one.

By shifting into a slower, more attentive state, we also have the opportunity to be able to see our loved one in a more honest way. In her recent book, *Life Lessons,* renowned psychiatrist Elisabeth Kubler-Ross talks about the concept of being able to see people in *the present,* not encumbered with a memory of what they were, nor in hope of what they might be in the future, but as they are *right now.*

More than a half-century earlier, in 1949, novelist Charles Yale Harrison suffered a life-threatening heart attack, which left him bedridden for nearly four months. Documenting his physical and emotional recovery in *Thank God for My Heart Attack,* he wrote:

Lying there, I thought of the human relationships I intended to strengthen and the meaningless and footling things that I would end. Trying to find the red thread of significance in my life, my mood toward everyone and everything was understanding, and, finally ... sympathy.[1]

Finding that point of sympathy and acceptance of your loved ones in their present state is a great blessing for you, for them, and for your relationships.

MaryKay's Story

That lesson came to me like peeling an onion, revealing itself one layer at a time until I came to the heart of it while coping with my sister's illness. MaryKay was diagnosed with breast cancer on June 10, 1996. The days that preceded the dreaded diagnosis were filled with mounting horror as hope slipped through our fingers. The lump she discovered could have been a benign cyst. The mammogram cast doubt on this slender hope, which the subsequent needle biopsy ruled out. The darkness closed in when the diagnosis was confirmed and the mastectomy was scheduled.

Because our mother had died of breast cancer in 1975, MaryKay's process held a dreadful déjà vu, which she struggled to overcome. I remember her saying, "This is not a death sentence. It's merely a speed bump in the road of life." The whole family and her friends rallied 'round that battle cry as she recovered from the surgery and then suffered through six months of chemotherapy. The process was viewed as being a short-term period of inconvenience—the speed bump on the road of her fast-paced life. She had to slow down, but this was not going to bring her to a full halt.

While I fully supported her in her speed-bump campaign,

she and I agreed that we needed to have a higher level of communication than we'd had with Mom, whose initial cancer diagnosis occurred in 1964 when my sister and I were teenagers. Our parents chose to limit what they told us in the belief that it would spare us unnecessary stress. Unfortunately, an unintended consequence of that decision was to quite literally keep my sister and me in the dark.

MaryKay wanted to shine more light on her process, so we talked about what it would be like to have full communication where we could all discuss our questions and fears and share our feelings. At the time of her diagnosis, she was fifty years old and my partner in running a small real estate development firm in Southern California. Our "staff" included our dad and her husband, Chuck. She was active in a variety of charitable organizations and busy with the rigors of raising their teenage son, Andrew. We all agreed that thorough communications would be a very good thing indeed, and so when she went through her surgery and subsequent chemo, we all talked a lot. Let me note here that Andrew tended to opt out of this extensive communication, which is normal behavior for any teenager, but especially for a boy whose mother has breast cancer. I believe he was very uncomfortable talking about his mother's breast.

However, while there was a lot more discussion about the disease and its treatment, there was still a pervasive sense that this was really just a brief episode to be gotten through and that life would return to utterly normal as soon as it was over. We continued to make our very bad jokes about plucking each other's chin hairs when we were in our nineties and living next door to each other in a rest home.

MaryKay's last chemotherapy treatment was in December of 1996. As she began to recover her strength, our father was diagnosed with non-Hodgkin's lymphoma, which was a recurrence of his 1991 bout with testicular cancer. And so the family effortlessly downshifted into the same medical support system while he underwent chemo and radiation treatments.

My dad, my sister, and I worked together in running our small real estate development company. During this period, we were in the process of emerging from some major financial disasters brought on by the Southern California real estate recession of the nineties. To lose one team member for six months and then another created a burden at work for all of us. And yet, even this workload problem could be easily framed in terms of a temporary occurrence. We knew things would return to normal when the treatments were over, and both my father and sister struggled into the office during their days of chemo to contribute what they could to our business.

It was so painful to see them in such depleted physical condition from the effects of the chemo and radiation, forcing themselves to come to the office and contribute to the family business. I recognize now that for them, being able to work at all was a blessing. Be prepared to see similar behavior in your patients. If they work, their job forms a large part of their identity. They may want to continue working in order to hold on to that piece of themselves, regardless of the state of their health. It's one of the ways they can keep hope active: seeing themselves in the future, continuing to hold their job after the medical journey is over and they have returned to health.

Family Experiences

By the time of MaryKay's initial diagnosis, she, Dad, and I had already acquired some skills and ideas for helping one another through these periods. After my mother died in 1975, my father, sister, and I became more involved in providing care for my father's parents.

Papa, Donald F. Shaw, had a history of heart problems, and Granny, Louisa Shaw, was suffering from advancing Parkinson's disease, so we needed to find home care for them and ensure that there was always a full schedule of these paid home helpers. Even with this level of in-home assistance, we still needed to be sure they were visited regularly and their non-medical needs were seen to.

My grandfather died suddenly of heart failure in 1979, and for the next six months, my grandmother was the complete focus of family attention until she died from pneumonia on the first day of 1980.

Shortly after my grandmother's death, my mother-in-law, Annette, was diagnosed with bone tumors, which were a recurrence of the cervical cancer that she'd been treated for five years earlier. She and my father-in-law, Darrell, lived in the same town as my grandparents, so in order to stay close, we drove an hour or went to their newly-built beach house two-and-a-half hours away. She was hospitalized for the last time just before Christmas 1980 and died a month later.

This was an exhausting period for me—trying to provide some care through personal contact with my loved ones who lived miles away across Southern California's choked freeway system, while caring for my own family and working full time as a journalist.

What I now realize is that this time of dealing with the deaths of these wonderful, important people in my life provided me with experiences that helped me later with my sister's and then my father's illnesses. The lessons that I've distilled for this book came from all of these experiences but are focused on the time I spent with my sister. My experience with my dad was less intensive for the simple reason that my stepmom, Claudette, was his primary caregiver, and I assumed a team member role in his care. For that reason, there will be fewer references to Dad's process than to MaryKay's.

The learning experiences offered by these family illnesses were interspersed with other medical crises experienced by friends:

- Betsy is a close friend who suffered a brain injury in a horse-riding accident. I actively participated in her recovery as one of a corps of volunteers who stayed with her in the hospital while she was in a coma and after she emerged from it.

- Paul and Jan were longtime family friends whose two daughters were key in my sister's care. Paul and my father were the closest of friends, beginning in their junior high school days. We lived two houses from one another during our growing up years, so the two sets of sisters were always together. Paul died of liver cancer in 1988, and Jan died in 1994 of lung cancer. Because their daughters, Ané de Nio and Joan McCormac, lived out of state, I filled in for them, staying close to their mother when they couldn't be with her.

- Sara, the dear woman who cared for my home and children for ten years while I was working, was diagnosed with cervical cancer and died three years later. It was in visits with Sara that I began to understand the value of spending time simply listening.

- Grant, our neighbor for twenty years, suffered from a variety of chronic conditions that eventually claimed his life. He was cared for by his wife, Inez, and from their experiences, I learned about the gift that visitors bring to a patient who is suffering and confined to a bed.

- Archie, a friend of just a few years duration but of a deep bond, announced one day at lunch that his prostate cancer had returned. He was a very successful venture capitalist who served on national non-profit boards of directors. He resigned from all of his worldly positions to focus on his family and friends in his final days. In doing so, he taught me about aligning your physical state with your spiritual and emotional well-being, even while being treated for a terminal illness.

All of these learning experiences coalesced in the late nineties, first with MaryKay's initial diagnosis and treatment for breast cancer and then with our dad's lymphoma and subsequent blood disorder. In the fall of 1997, Dad had been given a diagnosis of remission—we call it the "get-out-of-jail-free card" because there was no immediate further treatment prescribed—and I had decided to retire from the family real estate development firm in order to return to my first career as a writer.

December 19 of that year was a big day for all of us. It was our annual office Christmas lunch, and it was to be my last day in the family business. But MaryKay had a doctor's appointment that day to go over some test results because she'd been experiencing pain in her hip and lower back. The pain, we learned to our horror, was from bone tumors. Her cancer had returned.

And so, once again, the family shifted back into its medical crisis mode. I began my retirement, working part time to help MaryKay out at the office because she wasn't able to work full time herself. The chemotherapy she was undergoing was severe, and its side effects were acute. A few months after she began chemo, it was clear to all of us that I would need to work full time at our office so she could cope with her cancer treatments. Now we got into a new level of care.

As awful as the treatments were, for a while they seemed to be producing the desired results. But the good news was attended by a seemingly endless series of unanticipated new problems. New treatments were added that created new problems—radiation for brain lesions damaged her hearing, and an implant to deliver chemo to her brain became infected, leading to emergency brain surgery.

From Christmas 1997 to early March 1999, she put all her effort into overcoming her disease, as family and friends rallied to support her in a variety of ways—volunteers were organized to provide meals; our dear friend Ané de Nio took over as head caregiver, driving MaryKay to appointments, helping with the grocery shopping, and staying with her during the day when she was too frail to be left alone; and regular family meetings were held to make sure her needs were addressed. Her condition, however, slowly but steadily worsened.

In March of 1999, the cancer simply took over her body, and she was told that her condition was terminal. She died just before midnight on April 18, at home, with Mel Gutierrez, one of her professional caregivers, and me at her side.

Her final days were filled with blessings in the form of visits from family and friends. At first, Chuck and I thought about limiting the number of visits to one or two per day. However, we both quickly recognized that these wonderful people had come to express their love and say their good-byes. Because we had no way of knowing when the moment of her death would arrive, we didn't know whom to exclude. All of them were important in her life and she in theirs. We decided that even if there were four or five visitors in a day, that would be better than excluding someone who would perhaps never have the opportunity to share that last visit with her.

When patients are recovering from surgery or treatment, limiting visits is a wise move because it helps them preserve their energy for their recovery. When your patients are coming to the end of their days and are actively dying, there is no point in preserving energy. Of course, visits from friends and family need to be kept short. As caregivers, I hope you will be able to see the blessings to your patients in these visits.

One final thought to consider is your own energy level in accepting visitors. Take into account their needs to have a last visit with your patient, the patient's need to share these moments with family and friends, and then decide how much you can handle. Perhaps two visits a day are all you have energy for. I believe you'll find there are blessings to be found in the visits, and I hope you'll allow for as many as possible.

Looking for Light

What I learned from all these instances of illness or injury and the deaths that sometimes follow is that these times bring us to questions: What did I do (or he do or she do) to deserve this? Why can't we get out of this terrible situation? And when is this going to be over?

It's my experience that we use these questions like a shovel to dig ourselves deeper into the dark place that we've fallen into, and that makes the light just that much harder to find. Staying engaged with whatever the process is that the illness or injury has brought on is a huge challenge. But the ability to keep our eyes open in the darkness, to look for the light—because it is there—is a great blessing to be found, the gift that ultimately affirms life itself.

Rabbi Ben Kamin writes of the larger meaning of these blessings.

> A passage in *Gates of Prayer,* a prayer book of Reform Juda-ism, has always made sense to me: "The Psalmist said that in his affliction he learned the law of God. And in truth, grief is a great teacher, when it sends us back to serve and bless the living. We learn how to counsel and comfort those who, like ourselves, are bowed with sorrow. We learn when to keep silence in their presence, and when a word will assure them of our love and concern."[2]

For those of us who are caregivers, there is great weight in being such an intimate part of the patient's life-threatening experience or long-term care. There are an estimated fifty-four million adult Americans who are providing some level of care to a loved one, according to The National Family Caregivers Association (NFCA). These free caregiving services offered by family and friends are worth an estimated $196 billion a year. The American Association of Retired People (AARP) surveyed twenty-three hundred people between the ages of forty-five and fifty-five to find out how many of them were caregivers. The study found that on average 32 percent were providing care for another family member. That care is being provided against a backdrop of other demands—jobs, spouses and children, and keeping homes.

Don't underestimate the stress levels that being a care-giver generates, because it can make the darkness feel as if it is utterly without light. And it is dangerous not only to your emotional and spiritual well-being but to your health as well. A study written up in the *Journal of the American Medical Association,* begun in 1999, followed caregivers giving care to dementia patients. This group was studied because the caregivers were providing the care by themselves, with no outside assistance, and they were all over the age of sixty. Both characteristics—being over sixty and being a sole caregiver—are common among spouses caring for dementia patients. The medical team found that these caregivers experienced a 63 percent increase in mortality risk. That risk level is in the realm of people who are long-term smokers.[3]

The blessing is that medical science is just now beginning to take into account this and similar studies. The results are leading to assessment standards as well as treatment plans and programs, especially for the caregivers, recognizing that they can become disabled or mortally ill from the stress of the work they've taken on.

As you and your loved one find your way through this medical process, you will come to recognize that it is combined with larger emotional and spiritual issues as well. In that context, there are plenty of ordinary, seemingly commonplace blessings to be shared. They can be found in doing small things for the patient.

Whether you're being supportive through active listening; providing simple pleasures; going to doctors' appointments as a team member; volunteering with meals, housework, or babysitting; finding meaningful ways to be with your loved one; or seeking outside support, you're giving and receiving these wonderful blessings every day. These small ways of showing your love and caring shine light on both those who give and those who receive them.

Retired surgeon Bernie S. Siegel wrote of blessings in his book *Love, Medicine, and Miracles* when he described the effect of a serious illness on caregivers and patients as "a unique and difficult experience, not just a diagnosis that one prescribed treatment for."[4]

He's absolutely on target when he mentions that it's a difficult experience, which is a reality sometimes at odds with the expectations of the patient and their caregiver. Thanks to movies and television, we're conditioned to expect patients to be noble in their suffering and caregivers to be endlessly supportive and selfless. The reality is that your experiences won't always look like that, if they ever do at all. People who are seriously ill or injured don't feel well—or noble—and there are likely to be times when their behavior will reflect how ill they feel. Likewise, caregivers can get burned out or become overwhelmed, and their behavior will reflect their emotional state too.

Pain can be the source of problems between you and your loved one. Severe, ongoing pain is very debilitating—it literally sucks the energy out of the patient. It may cause your loved one to become inwardly focused and to shut down in terms of relating to others—you included. If that happens, you may feel left out in the darkness. When you experience that kind of loss of intimacy with your loved one, over time, it can lead you to feel burned out. I know from personal experience (a herniated disk in my lower spine that made walking almost impossible and left me bedridden for more than a month) that pain makes it very difficult to concentrate, to the point that even simple conversations become burdensome.

Someone who's hurting, and has been for some time, generally just wants to be left alone; he or she also can be angry and extremely difficult to be with, impossible to please. Try to keep in mind that when you encounter this situation, your loved one isn't rejecting you as a person; they simply need to find a way to cope with their pain.

The sixteen months between MaryKay's diagnosis of the cancer's recurrence and her death were just as Dr. Siegel described—unique and difficult; dark times indeed for all of us. But within those days of hope, followed by frustration and disappointment, there were moments of clarity about the lessons life and death have to teach all of us, lessons both great and small.

As we put into practice all that we had learned in the past about caring for someone who is seriously ill, we were also gaining new insights about ourselves as individuals and as family members, in the ways we found to connect with my sister and her struggle with her disease and growing disability. At the same time, on a higher level, we were given the opportunity to be able to see the transcendent meaning of an individual life, one of the greatest blessings in a time of darkness. Ultimately, that is the true meaning of light in a time of darkness. It's about giving and receiving love in the grief over your loved one's suffering, the ultimate gift that one human being can give to another.

Henri Nouwen, the late Catholic priest and spiritual writer, saw this level of blessing as a special form of celebration:

> Celebration is possible only through the deep realization that life and death are never found completely separate. Celebrations can really come about only where fear and love, joy and sorrow, tears and smiles can exist together. Celebration is the acceptance of life in a constantly increasing awareness of its preciousness.[5]

Seven centuries earlier, Jalal ad-Din Rumi, the Islamic poet and mystic, voiced this same principle:

> I saw grief drinking a cup of sorrow and called out, "It tastes sweet, does it not?" "You've caught me," grief answered, "and you've ruined my business, how can I sell sorrow when you know it's a blessing?"[6]

LESSON TWO:
THE EMOTIONAL IMPACT

Thanksgiving 1996

Thanksgiving was horrible. MaryKay was so sick and insisted on coming to the dinner that I gave for the family. She could barely stand to be at the dinner table, she was so nauseated by the food. Brave try, but I resented that. *Why didn't she stay home or flake out on the couch?* I kept thinking. *Why is she sitting here at the table, wincing at the food?* (Which, by the way, I'd spent two days lovingly preparing.) Again, it was get through it, pretend all is normal, and don't say you can't do it. "Don't look at it, don't touch it, and by the way, how are *you*, so you won't have to focus on me." It's how this family does this. I think another name for it might be denial.

W hile you are learning to adjust to the physical impact of your patients' medical conditions, you, as well as they, will be reeling from the emotional side effects of the new circumstances. The emotional impact is a significant portion of your experience as a caregiver and your loved one's experience as a patient. Understanding what the process is and how it will play out in both of your lives will go a long way to helping both of you cope with not only the emotional process but the medical process as well.

In the sixties, Dr. Elisabeth Kubler-Ross, a psychiatrist, began an unprecedented study of terminally ill patients at the University of Chicago Billings Hospital. Dr. Kubler-Ross and her medical students did something unthinkable at the time— they talked to the dying about their end-of-life experiences. Her findings, published in 1969 in her groundbreaking book *On Death and Dying*, have substantially changed the way in which American medicine treats people with terminal and life-threatening illnesses and serious injuries. Since then, her findings have become widely recognized to apply to people in a variety of traumatic circumstances, not just to those who are dying.

Central to her discoveries were the stages she observed all of her patients pass through as they processed the news of their impending deaths: denial, anger, bargaining, depression, and acceptance. In revisiting the five stages thirty years after her original book, Dr. Kubler-Ross illustrated her concept using the loss of a contact lens:

- *Denial*—I can't believe I dropped it!
- *Anger*—Darn it, I should have been more careful.
- *Bargaining*—I promise if I find it this time, I will be much more careful in the future.
- *Depression*—I am so sad that I lost it, now I will have to buy another.
- *Acceptance*—It's okay, I was bound to lose a contact someday. I'll order a new one in the morning.[1]

Since 1969, there have been a host of studies and papers from other disciplines in which the same five stages have been seen in *all* traumatic events of human life—loss of a job, end of a relationship, and even a move from one home to another. Psychiatrist M. Scott Peck, in his book *Denial of the Soul,* notes that "although Dr. Kubler-Ross didn't quite realize it at the time she wrote *On Death and Dying,* she had outlined stages that we go through anytime we make a significant psycho-spiritual growth step at any point during our lives."[2] In her most recent book, *Life Lessons,* Dr. Kubler-Ross does indeed acknowledge that the five stages "can be applied to our losses in life, whether big or small, permanent or temporary."[3]

I have seen these emotions at work in myself in all of my experiences with illness in my family and in times when other crises occurred. In reflecting on it, it seems to me that the reason the five stages show up at these other traumatic moments is that these other times represent little deaths—ending a relationship, an identity created by a job, or a time spent in a given neighborhood and home.

Every one of these events, especially an actual physical death, is followed by the unknown. Where do we go after we die? Who will love me now that I'm divorced? What will I do for a living? I may even know where my new home is, but the questions still remain about how I'll fit into the new neighborhood and what the details of my life will be like. The five stages ultimately enable us to release the old life and accept the new one, with all of its unknown aspects.

In a time of illness or injury, the *little death* aspect of the circumstances looms large. If the condition is chronic, such as with MS or kidney disease, or with a disabling injury, then the *death* is of the patient's previous lifestyle. Some level of their previous physical activity will be curtailed, and they may even be forced to change their living arrangements—another *little death*—to accommodate their new circumstances. The unknowns seem endless in terms of knowing what life will look like in the new system.

Dementia, such as Alzheimer's disease, brings a devastating double *death*, first in the loss of memory and personality before the patient succumbs to the disease. If the diagnosis is of a potentially life-threatening disease, such as cancer— as opposed to an actual terminal diagnosis—then the *death* is potential but also immediate. A patient who's facing removal of a diseased organ, in fact, is dealing with the *death* of that part of him or herself. If the cancer is being treated with radiation, there's a loss of bone marrow. Chemo brings on a temporary but very real loss of body hair.

All of these events trigger the five stages and can leave the patient questioning what his or her future will be like. Will my hair ever grow back? Will I be the same person I was before this started? Will I ever be normal again?

Those questions raised in a patient's mind are like a rock dropped into a quiet pond that sends expanding rings of ripples out to touch the closest family and friends, who may ask themselves the same kinds of questions—What will my relationship be like with my husband now? How will our family handle this illness/injury financially? The little deaths will affect this inner circle of friends and family as well as the patient.

A significant feature of the five stages, according to Dr. Kubler-Ross, is that patients do not move in a neat orderly progression from one to the next. She also discovered that patients generally do not remain permanently in any phase, including acceptance, once they've achieved that state. She believed—and my personal experiences reinforce—that we move through these stages constantly, with varying degrees of intensity, sometimes cycling back to one we've already passed through.

The first four stages—denial, bargaining, anger, and

depression—tend to be roadblocks to action, so both patients and caregivers need to be aware of them when they are taking place. Acceptance is a good place to be, but it's not always possible to remain in that state. When my dad was struggling with his cancer, his life reached a plateau in which the treatments, while draining for him, seemed to steady his health. He wasn't well, but he wasn't worsening, and so we all finally found a point of acceptance that the blood transfusions and chemo would be a way of life for him. However, as soon as his health worsened, even slightly, I realized I was once again bouncing around through the other four emotional stages. As Dr. Kubler-Ross notes, "These [the five stages] will last for different periods of time and will replace each other or exist at times side by side."[4]

One reason for the recycling through the various stages, according to Dr. Peck, is the discomfort that each of the stages—except acceptance—brings with it. He sites depression as an example. "When they hit it, [depression] is so painful that they do not know they can work through it, so they retreat back into the earlier stages, particularly denial."[5]

As a result of her study, Dr. Kubler-Ross came to believe that effective and compassionate communication between physician and patient—and between the medical team, the patient, and their family and close friends—was an important component of the treatment process. It's a two-sided coin. There needs to be a high level of communication among all concerned about the patient and with the patient. And there needs to be a clear understanding of the five stages. For the most positive of outcomes in terms of the diagnosis, treatment, and ongoing life of the patient, these two processes need to function hand in hand.

As I mentioned, there was a great contrast between my experiences with my mother's cancer and my sister's. With Mom, the information about her condition, prognosis, and treatments was withheld to keep from upsetting my sister and me. My parents based this decision on the fact that we were in our junior and senior years of high school, respectively, and needed to be left undisturbed to study. In MaryKay's time of dealing with cancer, we talked as much as she could about her circumstances—more in the initial diagnosis and treatment phases, somewhat less in the recurrence. Still, my experience agrees with Dr. Kubler-Ross; knowing what's happening and having the ability to express feelings are extremely important to the patient and circle of caregivers.

The Five Stages
DENIAL

Nearly everyone touched by a medical crisis does start with some form of denial, which focuses on the central question of how such a thing could be, with the resulting thought that there must be some mistake. This is a common response to a medical crisis, and it denies the reality of the situation. That doesn't make denial a bad thing. Denial is a necessary coping mechanism, especially in the early stages of learning that someone has a serious illness.

With my sister's discovery of a lump in her breast, neither she nor the rest of the family immediately leaped ahead to the conclusion that it was a malignancy. Instead, we engaged in a level of denial by assuming the most benign outcome for each of the successive tests until the final diagnosis was given. Even at that point, the denial took the form of focusing on the future recovery with MaryKay's statement that the diagnosis of cancer was "just a speed bump on the road of life."

In *On Death and Dying,* Dr. Kubler-Ross described denial this way:

> I emphasize this strongly, since I regard it as a healthy way of dealing with the uncomfortable and painful situation with which some of these patients have to live for a long time. Denial functions as a buffer after unexpected shocking news, allows the patient to collect himself and, with time, mobilize other, less radical defenses.[6]

More than thirty years later, Dr. Kubler-Ross expanded on her understanding of the role of denial, adding the thought that denial is a beautiful grace that enables us to gather ourselves emotionally, intellectually, and physically to deal with a pending death of some portion of ourselves.[7]

However, denial can also be a detriment when it persists or takes an extreme form. Patients who won't take medications or won't get needed therapy or treatment because they don't believe they're ill are in a dangerous form of denial. Dr. Kubler-Ross documented a case of a patient who endlessly sought second opinions, searching for a physician who would give her the diagnosis she wanted to hear—that she wasn't ill at all. In these cases, she notes that physicians, family, and friends can be most helpful if they support beneficial behaviors, such as taking medication, but don't concentrate on forcing the patient to drop this strongly held denial. They may be hanging on to it because it's impossible for them to face the reality of their circumstance.

At a support group, I met a woman, Mrs. A, whose husband was in denial of his diagnosis of Alzheimer's disease. He had prohibited the family from discussing it with anyone and refused to see the neurologist who'd given him the initial diagnosis. "We are losing precious time, and he won't accept any treatment," Mrs. A. tearfully told the group. Group members were sympathetic but could offer no magic advice for getting the husband to release his denial and start treatment to help slow the inevitable progress of the disease. They advised her to keep coming to the support group and use stress-reducing activities such as exercise and prayer to care for herself while he refused care for himself. They also recommended that she keep telling him what she wanted, which was for him to get treatment. "Keep talking to him about it," they told her. "If nothing else, you'll feel better because you know you did all that was possible."

ANGER

Denial—which is also expressed by family and friends—is "usually a temporary defense and will soon be replaced by partial acceptance," according to Dr. Kubler-Ross.[8] This partial acceptance is replaced with feelings of anger, rage, envy, and resentment. The question becomes: Why? Why me? Why my loved one? Why now? Why not someone else?

Dr. Kubler-Ross notes that this is a very difficult stage for those around the patient—their support group of family and friends, as well as the medical team.

> [The anger] is displaced in all directions and projected onto the environment at times almost at random...What else would we do with our anger, but let it out on...people who rush busily around only to remind us that we cannot even stand on our two feet anymore. People who order unpleasant tests and prolonged hospitalization with all its limitations, restrictions, and costs, while at the end of the day

they can go home and enjoy life. People who tell us to lie still so that the infusion or transfusion does not have to be restarted, when we feel like jumping out of our skin to be doing something in order to know that we are still functioning on some level.[9]

In her later book, Dr. Kubler-Ross drew a parallel between denial and anger as both being potentially beneficial. As she noted about the grace of denial, she also points out that anger in the proper portions and at the right time and place can be beneficial, citing "studies [that] have shown over and over again that angry patients live longer," possibly because they have learned to express their anger and use it to demand better care.[10]

Still, it doesn't make the caregiver's life any easier being around anger that's flying in all directions. From an experience with my dad when he'd been hospitalized in 1991, I learned that my best response was to let him have his anger without getting caught up in it myself.

He'd been hospitalized with an adverse reaction to radiation treatments. He was angry at himself for not following his doctor's orders about what and what not to eat and drink during these treatments and at the world in general, the kind of anger Dr. Kubler-Ross describes. When he turned it on the medical technician who showed up with a wheelchair to take him for some tests, I couldn't stand it. It was pointless to tell him how rude he was being. I simply left, vowing to limit visits with him when he was in that state. I couldn't change his anger, but I didn't need to expose myself to it either. The anger usually dissipates, according to Dr. Kubler-Ross, when patients have opportunities to express their feelings.

It is ironic that having outlined this stage so thoroughly, Dr. Kubler-Ross found herself in it as a result of having suffered a series of debilitating strokes in the late nineties. She spoke from personal experience in *Life Lessons* when she wrote about being berated for being angry over her physical condition. "It's as if [my circle of intimates] loved my stages but didn't like me being in one of them. But those who stayed with me allowed me to be, not judging me or my anger, and that helped me to dissipate it."[11]

Caregivers are also susceptible to this emotional phase. Check yourself when you are angry. What's the true source of your anger? Is it the inattentiveness of the doctor's receptionist, or is it the fact that you're in the doctor's office at all in the role of caregiver? The challenge for caregivers is to determine if the anger they're experiencing is from the emotional stage underlying this significant change in their lives or if it's generated by their patients' behaviors.

I call anger that's in response to a behavior one of the "ugly faces of caregiving," because sometimes it can lead us into feelings of guilt. One woman in a caregiver support group I led came to the group very angry with her husband. "He refuses to acknowledge his disability and won't leave early enough for an appointment. I am fed up with constantly running late for everything," she told us. In addition to the anger, based on her husband's behavior, she was feeling guilty because "He's sick, I'm healthy, and I shouldn't get mad at him."

The anger-guilt cycle can cause caregivers to focus even more exclusively on their patients' needs, to the exclusion of their own well-being. One way to deal with this issue is to talk it out with a friend or a support group, or journal it out. Getting it out in conversation or down on paper is a good way to recognize what the feelings are so that they don't become your primary motivator.

BARGAINING

The bargaining phase is usually the briefest. If the anger is based on the question of why, then bargaining is a way to try to influence the answer. Sometimes, when the answer is that the patient believes he or she deserved it in some way—even if it was "just the luck of the draw"—then bargaining is one response. It's like punishing a child, even if they don't believe they deserve the punishment. After the initial outburst, the child may come back with a bargain—if I put out the trash for the next month, will you cut short the time I'm grounded?

Dr. Kubler-Ross notes that an intrinsic part of this stage is that a promise is made for a goal to be obtained. For example, I might promise God that I'd go to church every day in exchange for a benign diagnosis of my sister's breast lump.

Bargaining is an emotional response that is probably as old as humanity itself. Psalm 79, which was written some 2,500 years ago, demonstrates our willingness to strike bargains with God to get what we want. This particular psalm was written after the Babylonians had invaded Judah, captured Jerusalem, sacked the temple, and carried most of the inhabitants off to slavery in Babylon. Here's the psalmist's attempt at making a bargain with God:

> Return sevenfold into the bosom of our neighbors
> the taunts with which they taunted you, O Lord!
> Then we your people, the flock of your pasture,
> will give thanks to you forever;
> from generation to generation we will recount your praise.
>
> Psalm 79:12–13

With you and your patient, you can expect this phase to pass within days or at most a week or two. It's simply a matter of the reality of the medical situation moving you beyond this phase. Bargaining is difficult to hang on to when treatments are commencing. At that point, either tacitly or openly, the reality of the circumstances has to be acknowledged by you both. For instance, someone may bargain with God for there to have been a mistake and that their test results really belong to some other patient. Obviously, this won't hold up as the patient's surgery is performed or other treatment commenced.

For caregivers, bargaining can be a helpful tool, or it can be an impediment to giving the care that's needed. A woman new to a support group for Alzheimer's caregivers told the group members that she knew her husband would recover because she was going to church every day and praying for him. She had no need of information about the disease because soon he would not be afflicted with it, she said. You can see how this woman's bargaining was interfering with her care of her husband.

On the other hand, caregivers may intentionally use bargaining as a means of getting their patients to take medications or show up for medical appointments or therapy. It can sometimes be like bribing a small child who doesn't want to go to the doctor by offering an ice cream cone afterwards.

As in the case of the woman whose husband had Alzheimer's, bargaining is another emotional stage that can freeze caregivers and prevent them from taking the action needed to support their patients. *Why do all that work when my bargaining is going to lead to his or her recovery?* As with anger, I recommend that you listen to your spoken and unspoken thoughts. Are you offering a "deal" to get your patients to do what you know they need to do to support their recovery? If so, that is helpful to the medical journey you're on together. On the other hand, if you are still trying to make a bargain with God to miraculously heal your loved one, then you're stuck in this emotional stage. Ask yourself if your attitude is helping or hurting your patient. If you're honest, you can see when you're bargaining to deny the reality of your circumstances, and I'm hopeful you will be able to end this phase quickly and get on with the caregiving work that your patient really needs from you.

DEPRESSION

This is the stage at which the darkness will seem the deepest and the light farthest away from you and your loved one. This is probably the hardest stage to work through, and it is definitely the one where the tears will flow most freely. And because it is the most emotionally demanding, it is the one from which you and your loved one are most likely to retreat into an earlier stage, usually anger or denial.

Depression is the stage where you or your loved one can *bottom out* by getting in touch with all of the emotions around the medical crisis—not just the anger but the fear of the unknown and the sorrow over losses that may result from the medical circumstance. But thoroughly experiencing this phase comes with a great reward, and that's the ability, once the hard work has been done, to move beyond it and into a state of acceptance. There can be a very marked shift from the darkness of depression to the light of acceptance.

Dr. Kubler-Ross describes two types of depression, both of which relate to losses resulting from the medical condition. The first type is directly related to the medical condition. A very understandable example is the depression suffered by women with breast cancer who undergo mastectomies. They will grieve the loss of their breasts and perhaps the resulting loss of self-esteem for feeling they may no longer be as feminine as they once were. Just because there are ways of compensating for physical losses—in this example, implants or prostheses—that doesn't mean a patient in this circumstance isn't going to experience depression at the loss.

Mary Susan Herczog, in a yearlong series of articles in the *Los Angeles Times,* wrote about discovering a lump in her breast, which she dismissed as being a cyst. After all, she'd been diagnosed with cysts, which had been drained a few weeks before the new lumps appeared. She "continued to dismiss it for a few weeks until it grew to more than the size of a peach pit and turned very hard.

"When a lump turned up in my armpit, I knew. Or rather, suspected. Because there are things you don't allow yourself to think," she wrote.

She went to her radiologist who took a biopsy on Thursday and told her to call on Monday. She and her husband spent the weekend telling themselves that it would turn out to be nothing. They supported this hope with the facts of Mary's life—she never drank, smoked, did drugs, or drank coffee, tea, or soda.

"I even exercise regularly. And I eat sort of low-fat, except when I'm in New Orleans."

But on that following Monday, she was told the biopsy was "suspicious for cancer." A few days later, the cancer was confirmed and a treatment plan was made, involving months of chemotherapy, followed by a lumpectomy, radiation, and more chemo.

> You can spend a week thinking, "What if I have cancer, okay, so I'm going to lose my hair, which is bad, but I love hats, and I can explore my inner drag queen by wearing wigs" and other Pollyanna things. But actually hearing someone tell you that removing your breast is a possibility in your future … well, pass the Kleenex.[12]

Dr. Kubler-Ross says the second type of depression "does not occur as a result of a past loss, but is taking into account impending losses."[13] You can understand this *future loss* depression if you think in terms of dreams suddenly made unattainable by the medical condition. For instance, dialysis patients who may no longer be able to travel because of the regimens of treatment would suffer depression because they will never be able to take some trip that had been dreamed of for years. If they'd always wanted to go on a journey to the Holy Land and are now realizing this will never be possible, it's not helpful to try to cheer them up by explaining how expensive and dangerous such a trip would be and that they are better off not taking it.

It's important for loved ones who want to support the patient to be able to distinguish between the two. In the case of the depression about loss around the medical circumstance, patients need reassurance. The woman who has lost a breast needs to know from those she loves that in their eyes she is as feminine as she was before the surgery. In the second case, the patient doesn't need—nor probably want—cheering up. Your loved ones need to be allowed to express their sorrow over no longer being able to achieve one of their dreams. It is most helpful for family and friends to keep in mind that in the first type of depression, they can be most effective by offering their reassurances. Supporting a patient in this first type of depression, family and friends are the ones who do the most talking. In the second type, it is more effective to let the patients talk about their feelings of loss and having those feelings validated by family and friends.

The depression phase can be dangerous if it is deep and persistent. Dr. Nick Yaru, an orthopedic surgeon, said he literally lost his will to live in the depression that came after his diagnosis of prostate cancer. At one point, he attempted suicide. Fortunately, his life was saved, his cancer was successfully treated, and he eagerly returned to his medical practice. Equally fortunate for his patients, the experience changed Nick into the remarkably warm, caring physician he is today.

The point of Nick's story is that depression can be dangerous when it reaches this level. I strongly recommend that psychological therapy be obtained for a patient who drops into a deep and persistent depression.

If the illness or injury has a specific duration of treatments, as in radiation for cancer patients, then the depression may not occur until after the treatments are over. Selma Schimmel, founder of *The Group Room,* a radio talk show for cancer patients, suggests that when patients are no longer *doing something* they are left with a vacuum in which to deal with their emotions, and that empty space is where depression can occur.[14]

Regardless of the type of depression or when it occurs, it's not a stage that can be skipped or ignored. Dr. Peck strongly advocates for the necessity and rewards of doing the work of depression in order to reach acceptance. For him, that means confronting the depression and understanding its source and the emotions behind it—the fear and anger that have generated it. Only after Dr. Peck has done that work does he feel it's possible to reach a place of acceptance. For me, depression centers on grieving, and that is also hard work. It is easier to get through a day without the sorrow and tears of grief, but the alternative is to slip back into another stage, and the result is to miss gaining the stage of acceptance.

For the caregiver, depression can take a variety of forms. It can range from deep sadness and weeping to sleeplessness and constant fatigue. Loss of sex drive is part of it. When I was caring for my mother, there were sleepless, tear-filled nights, and I generally felt exhausted all the time. When I was caring for my grandmother, I sometimes felt like I simply could not get into my car and drive an hour or more to her house. I remember asking myself in these circumstances, "Why do I feel this way?" The answer, when I had the courage to confront it, was that these women who were so precious to me were dying, and I was powerless to change that fact. It is always painful to have to admit something like that, or even that your loved one's life—and yours—have changed permanently. But when you can confront that truth, you can find acceptance and with it a release from the depression that's weighing you down. I believe you will find yourself reenergized for the work of caregiving in this process.

ACCEPTANCE

Acceptance of the disease's presence in the patient's life, the reality of a debilitating injury, or even pending death, is the final stage, which is arrived at only in working through the earlier stages. This stage rests on the dual pillars of faith and trust. It is the place where patients are able to let go of the necessity of having specific results from their medical process, trusting that whatever the outcome, it is what is meant to be. Acceptance is a surrender to the higher power. Dr. Kubler-Ross cautions that "acceptance should not be mistaken for a happy stage."

Another way to look at this phase is to think of it in terms of alignment of all aspects of the patient's life—the physical with the emotional and spiritual. Ideally, this alignment can extend beyond your patients into their circle of other family and friends. If your patients are going to achieve that place of faith and trust, then it follows that those of you who are closest to them will have to be able to achieve that state too. When patients reach that place of faith and trust, it becomes necessary for those closest to them to find that same acceptance as well. Dealing with a life-threatening illness, a life-changing injury, or a chronic condition is difficult and demanding physically, emotionally and spiritually. But the struggle will seem much harder to the patients if those closest to them are still dealing with the other four emotional stages. In my example of the dialysis patient, it would mean that the patient and all of the members of the inner circle accept the new circumstances and no longer rage over the lost ability to travel. Acceptance means that not only is your loved one at peace with that fact but so are the rest of you; otherwise, there's no true alignment.

Acceptance is deeply woven into twelve-step recovery programs, especially in the motto "Let go and let God," which reflects the understanding that we can't—and don't need to— control the outcome and that we need to release that outcome to a higher power.

Dale A. Matthews, MD, wrote *The Faith Factor* to illustrate how scientifically valid studies consistently show the beneficial effect of faith on the lives of patients. He recounts the following story, which underscores how acceptance works for a patient:

Laura was a young woman who was dealing with a permanent physical disability as the result of a brain tumor. He asked her if she'd had any depression.

> "Yes, I have," she said, "but after you carry that burden for a while, you realize there's nothing you can do about it. Either you've got to hold on to it or let it go. So I let it go. I have my good days and my bad, and I decided to dwell on the good things and forget about the bad, since I can't do anything about the negative things in my life."[15]

For me, acceptance is simply that, ceasing to fight against what is happening. With any of my caregiving assignments, I would have days when I had not reached acceptance, and it all just seemed so impossible and painful, a real struggle on all fronts. When I finally became aware of the shifts in emotional states while taking care of MaryKay, I also became aware of a serenity that finally came over me, the serenity of acceptance. It wasn't that the work was any less painful or sad; it was that I finally could recognize that her condition wasn't going to change and that my job was to support her to the best of my ability. When I was no longer struggling against the reality of her cancer and could accept that it wasn't going to change, then I was able to offer her a higher level of energy and care.

GUILT AND HOPE

Dr. Kubler-Ross recognized that wrapped around the framework of the five stages were two seemingly opposing forces—hope and guilt. These two emotions are present in varying levels over time, functioning as a background setting to the work of the five stages, depending on each individual patient's emotional makeup and personal experience.

Guilt is the negative that can bring the work of the five stages to a halt, with the patients or the caregivers blaming themselves for the medical condition. Hope, on the other hand, is what keeps the patient and their loved ones moving forward. Retired surgeon Bernie S. Siegel writes of hope in his book *Love, Medicine and Miracles:* "When a doctor can instill some measure of hope, the healing process sometimes starts even before the treatment begins."[16] Hope is a necessary component not only through the process of treatment but also through the process of reaching acceptance. With either guilt or hope, it's important to know the degree to which these emotions color the process of reaching acceptance and how they can sidetrack it, in the case of guilt, or assist it, in the case of hope.

Dr. Kubler-Ross found guilt to be a common characteristic reaction seen often in families of people recently diagnosed with a serious illness, or even those who have suffered a serious injury. She noted in *On Death and Dying* that both patients and families who found themselves in this circumstance often reacted as if the medical circumstance were somehow their fault—they should have somehow kept their loved one safer, should have been able to prevent the onset of the illness in some way, or should have predicted the diagnosis earlier so treatment could have begun sooner with the possibility of a better outcome. If the caregiver or patient gets focused on these self-blaming recriminations, they are going to get stuck on a very dark, dead-end street that gives the illusion there's no way out. Movement through the five stages halts because the patients or their caregivers keep coming back to the issue of blame.

Acceptance is just that, acceptance of the medical condition as something that is a state of being—the heart condition, kidney failure, AIDS, stroke, Alzheimer's, or whatever the condition, *it is what it is*. Guilt over how it came into being won't change the fact of its existence and its impact on the patient's life. The thought that somehow your loved one's condition can be blamed on someone or something ignores the myriad of possibilities related to the cause of the illness or injury, the *fact* of the mystery of the medical crisis. Blame and regrets like these keep those who are engaging in this guilt loop in the darkness.

On the other hand, hope is the great gift of the process, regardless of the expected outcome. Dr. Kubler-Ross noted that in all five stages the patients she studied always had hope, the feeling that their condition must have some meaning and would pay off eventually if they could only endure it for a little while longer. "All our patients maintained a little bit of it and were nourished by it in especially difficult times."[17]

Dr. Siegel uses a motto from the book *Getting Well Again* by oncologist O. Carl Simonton and his psychologist wife, Stephanie Matthews: "In the face of uncertainty, there is nothing wrong with hope."[18]

Selma Schimmel, herself a former cancer patient, describes hope as being ever present for the thousands of cancer patients that she's encountered in her work on the radio show and as president of the foundation that supports it. She notes that the power hope carries is in allowing the patient and the caregiver to be in the moment rather than fretting over what may—or may not—happen next. It's the same quality that makes acceptance such a gift. Significantly, she points out that hope can only be fully present when fear and anger have been dealt with.

> [Hope is] empowering, calming, reassuring, and changing. Hope doesn't go away, although it transforms itself to adapt to one's situation and needs. Once you open up and stare down the feelings of fear and anger, you make room for hope. Hope lightens the load and helps you live in the moment, which is so much more meaningful than contemplating tomorrow.[19]

Hope, or the belief that the experience has a payoff, is different from optimism, which is the belief that all will be well in the end. Hope centers on the acceptance of the circumstances; optimism looks for the best possible outcome. Both are beneficial in terms of the patient's process through diagnosis and treatment.

My suggestion is that you always allow for optimism whenever possible, taking care to read cues given to you by your loved ones. If they are in a depressed state and see very little hope or cause for optimism, then having you come in with a Pollyanna outlook that all will be well will probably only increase the depths of their despair because you are not acknowledging their feelings at that moment.

When you don't necessarily want to echo their bleak out-look, you can engage in active listening skills. This is a system in which you can acknowledge your patients' emotional state and mirror it back to them—"I can see how you'd feel like this is hopeless. You're in a lot of pain, and you don't feel the treatments are working ... " This will also allow you a small space to share your thoughts—"I feel like I'm seeing a bit of improvement because yesterday you couldn't do what you can do today. I'm glad you're making a little bit of progress." Don't cram your optimism down their throats. Say it once and let go of it, unless they want to pick up on what you've offered. If they choose to open doors to that conversation, you can be willing to let them lead both of you through it.

Likewise, it can be the patients who are expressing hope and optimism while you, the caregivers, are seeing none. Again, you are there to support them, to let them set the agenda, not to force your mind-set onto them. So that may mean that when you're not feeling particularly hopeful, you are going to need to find a way to support your patient's optimism. Active listening can be a great tool to use in this circumstance too.

● ● ●

Even when you and your loved ones can achieve a high level of communication about your feelings and expectations for the treatment outcome, make no mistake that the process is still going to be a challenge. The emotional impact of your patients' medical condition is significant for you as well as them. The five stages of emotional processing apply to the patients *and* their closest circle of supporters.

Learning to accept the reality of the disease or injury is an extremely dynamic process. You as a caregiver, along with the patient, will be cycling through various stages in a somewhat random, not linear, manner. Denial may give way to anger that leads right back to denial rather than on to bargaining. Acceptance may be achieved, and then a development in the medical condition will send the patient back to an earlier stage. You and the patient aren't going to be cycling through the process in the same way. Understanding how this process works and what the stages look like for you, as well as for the patient, is a fundamental skill for supporting your loved one.

The treatment process is a journey along a winding path. The five stages and the presence of hope or guilt are part of the scenery that you have to pass through. Sometimes these emotions will function as signs that tell you where you are. This is not an easy journey, but like all trips, it has its own blessings in giving you the opportunity to see sights, meet people, and learn things you've not encountered before.

"The greatest lesson I've learned in life is you have to appreciate the moments in your life that are hard. You can't go run from adversity. You have to let it hit you straight in the face." Trent Dilfer, the quarterback of the Baltimore Ravens, was talking about his career setbacks prior to winning Superbowl XXXV, not a life-threatening illness. But what he had to say is a succinct summary of the lessons Dr. Kubler-Ross learned from her dying patients and that you have the opportunity to learn in caring for your loved one.

LESSON THREE:
THE CONNECTION OF MIND, BODY, AND SPIRIT

February 3, 1998

I am emotionally exhausted. No, I'm physically, spiritually, and emotionally exhausted. I seem to start every day by heaving a great sigh, as if expelling some air will make room for energy to flow in and restore me. My life is split between great joy in having the time and space to write again, even if it's just part time, and great grief in coming to grips with the fact that I'm losing my sister. Because of her illness and my need to support her in *any* way that I can, I am back doing the work that I basically dislike, and doing it because I feel compelled to. It all leaves me without reserves. It's not just physical and emotional—it's spiritual too. I'm exhausted in all realms. My prayer life is really blossoming. I'm swimming in deeper spiritual waters than ever before—which is wonderful! But that too is an energy drain.

Synergism is a term biologists use to explain the unexplainable, when two or more substances, organs, or organisms combine to achieve an effect that neither is capable of on its own.[1] It is a concept that was adopted as a buzzword in corporate America in the nineties to indicate a circumstance in which the sum totaled more than the component parts—two plus two equals five. It seems like such an intriguing idea until we try to apply it to ourselves as individual human beings.

For some of us, the synergism of the mind, body, and spirit connection is obvious. "Of course," we say. "Two plus two equals five, or six, or ten, or twenty. The sum depends on how lively the connection is among the parts." But for others, who hold a more mechanical view of the world and themselves in it, two plus two always equals four, never more, never less.

My experience—along with a growing body of scientific research—indicates the synergistic model is a more accurate depiction of human beings than the compartmentalized, mechanistic view is. There are countless books on this subject, which explore it in great depth. What I want to offer here are some basic ideas for you to incorporate as you and your loved ones deal with what may appear to you to be an experience limited to their physical condition. The level of recovery that you are hoping will be achieved is very much dependent on aligning and bringing to the recovery effort all the components of the self—the body with its mind and spirit. Retired surgeon Bernie S. Siegel frames the idea very well when he writes that "The issue is not about living forever and testing God, but utilizing all of the physical and emotional forces available for healing."[2]

It's not too difficult to define what I mean by the body or the physical aspect of a human being. We can experience it with all of our senses. We can touch it, hear it, see it, smell it, and even taste it. It is the most real because it is the most obvious part of a human being. But as our bodies are themselves made up of various organs and limbs, our total self—our being—is made up of component parts as well. When we get to the other two—the mind, or intellect, and the spirit, or soul—then it gets a bit trickier because of our fondness for experiencing and describing things in physical terms.

If the body is the most physical aspect of a human being, the thing we can most readily detect with our senses, then the mind is halfway between physical and nonphysical. The dictionary defines mind as: "The human consciousness that originates in the brain and is manifested especially in thought, perception, feeling, will, memory, or imagination."[3] We know where it originates, in the chemical reactions within the brain—again something we can detect with our sense of sight by looking at various kinds of brain scans while the organ is doing its work—but there is no physical presence to the product that the mind turns out. The results of that physical effort are nonphysical in nature. We can't use our senses to perceive the mind in the same way we can use them to perceive the body.

The spirit, as something that is completely nonphysical, is at the opposite end of the physicality scale from the body. Interestingly, it is defined as "that which is traditionally believed to be the vital principle or animating force within living beings" and "that which constitutes one's unseen, intangible being."[4] In other words, the spirit, the part of us that is nonphysical, is by definition that which gives life to the physical aspect of ourselves.

Medicine's View of the Connection

While it seems so important in our culture to be able to describe our world in physical terms, we have these significant portions of ourselves that are not at all physical in nature. Yet none of us would describe ourselves without mention of our nonphysical aspects—our personalities, our character, our emotions, our imagination, our sense of humor, or our intelligence. How we are in the world, how we behave, is governed by these nonphysical aspects of ourselves, so they are very much worth paying attention to in your time of medical crisis.

The medicine practiced by ancient cultures, such as the Egyptian, Greco-Roman, and mediaeval Christian, all took into account the unseen aspects of a patient's totality when treating an illness. Those unseen components were viewed as being as important as the physical symptoms. The same was true of many of the non-European indigenous cultures that predated the conquests of the past five centuries.

Dr. Siegel notes that Hippocrates, the ancient Greek who is the father of modern medicine, said he would rather know what sort of person has a disease than what sort of disease a person has:

> Neglect of the mind-body link by technological medicine is actually a brief aberration when viewed against the whole history of the healing art. In traditional tribal medicine and in Western practice, from its beginning in the work of Hippocrates, the need to operate through the patient's mind has always been recognized. Until the nineteenth century, medical writers rarely failed to note the influence of grief, despair, or discouragement on the onset and outcome of illness, nor did they ignore the healing effects of faith, confidence, and peace of mind.[5]

The shift by science and medicine to reliance solely on physical evidence dates from the seventeenth century. It was a time of revolutionary changes in thinking started by Francis Bacon and expanded upon when French philosopher Rene Descartes (1596–1650) published *Discourse on Method,* which established the scientific method of inquiry based on systematic doubt. Descartes's idea was to start with a question then use a physical process—observation of data—from which an answer could be postulated. The Cartesian model has been the underpinning of all scientific advancement for the past 350 years.

> In his discourse, Descartes wrote that instead of the "speculative philosophy of the schools" mankind should be able to understand "the forces and action of fire, water, air...as distinctly as we understand the mechanical arts of our craftsmen...we can use these forces in the same way for all purposes for which they are appropriate, and so make ourselves the masters and possessors of nature. And this is desirable...mainly for the preservation of health, which is undoubtedly the principal good and foundation of all other good things in this life."[6]

Descartes's scientific method was further refined by eighteenth-century thinkers like philosopher David Hume and physician/philosopher/sociologist John Locke who eliminated non-observable phenomena, such as spirituality, from being in the realm of the scientifically provable. The ideas of these philosophers pushed western civilization further down the road that held if something isn't physically observable, it probably doesn't exist.

Ironically, Descartes, who started this revolution in scientific thought, had used his method of systematic doubt to *prove* the existence of God as part of what is now called Cartesian dualism, because it made room for both the physically observable and the nonphysical, which he labeled "thinking substance."[7]

Physician Larry Dossey says the rationalistic scientific attitude really blossomed in Western medicine in the last third of the nineteenth century.

[This era] encompasses the discovery and practice of therapies that largely dominate Western medicine today—drugs,
surgery, radiation, and so on … According to these "laws,"
the entire universe, including the body, is a vast clockwork
that functions according to deterministic, causal principles … This means that in [this era] the effects of mind and
consciousness were considered of secondary importance, *if
of any importance at all.*[8]

Dr. Dossey says that outlook began to change after World
War II into a practice of medicine that incorporates the holistic approach integrating the mind, body, and spirit connection,
as witnessed by the development of techniques such as biofeedback to help control bodily responses such as perception
of pain. Although he notes that this new era is still characterized by a great deal of official skepticism about the integrated
approach to medicine, he goes on to say that he believes medicine is at the edge of a far broader understanding of the use of
the mind for healing purposes.[9]

The Connection in Healing

So what do the ruminations of this group of philosophers,
scientists, and physicians mean to you and your patient? Primarily, it means the medical system that will be treating your
loved one is not likely to make use of the understanding that
well-being is based on the complex and intricate linkage of the
body to mind and spirit.

Physician Dale Matthews notes that "doctors live in a
world completely dominated by Cartesian philosophy, trained
to think only in terms of what can be empirically proved in
the laboratory. The prospect of discussing … subjective spiritual experiences … makes many doctors feel uncomfortable."[10]

Likewise, physicians, for the most part, are equally uncomfortable in considering a course of treatments that would harness the unseen power of the mind along with drugs and other commonly used traditional therapies.

Yet both Dr. Dossey and Dr. Matthews can cite numerous scientific studies and have a wide range of anecdotal experiences that support the concept that our health and well-being is not limited to a function of our physical selves but of an interaction between body, mind, and spirit. Another medical advocate of the connection is Dr. Siegel, who uses emotions and imagery to work with his surgery patients.

> We don't yet understand all the ways in which brain chemicals are related to emotions and thoughts, but the salient point is that our state of mind has an immediate and direct effect on our state of body ... Emotions and imagery ... are two ways we can get our minds and bodies to communicate with each other.[11]

An analogy that puts this concept of the mind-body-spirit linkage in common terms can be useful in understanding the necessity of drawing on all three aspects of the self.

Best-selling psychologist Wayne W. Dyer urges us to think of the body as the "garage in which you park your soul."[12] "Treat your body like a guest who visits and then must leave ... Honor it, welcome it, and allow it to take its course ... Be in awe of every inch of it."[13] If the body is the home and the soul is the guest that stays there, then the mind provides the systems that make the home work, that open and close the doors to keep it safe in the world, and that ensures the pipes have running water and the electrical lines carry power to turn on the lights and heat the space.

The first concern, I believe, is to have all three elements

working together. An illness or injury has an overwhelm-ingly physical nature to it, and so the tendency is to focus on that alone and ignore the mind and spirit. If ants invade your kitchen, you don't hustle everyone out of the house and shut off the power and water, do you? More likely, you'll get every-one in the house to pitch in and help, using all of the resources the home provides to get the ants cleaned out of the kitchen. When you are facing a serious illness, why approach the cir-cumstances any differently? Use all the resources that can be brought to bear on the problem—mental and spiritual as well as physical. How can you do that? You and your patient can engage your minds by learning as much as possible about the disease that is causing the crisis. Bring your soul or spiritual side into the caregiving by praying with and for your patient, and with and for the medical team.

The second issue is one of priorities. Sometimes in focus-ing on the physical nature of an illness, mind and spirit aren't ignored but are assigned lesser roles, usually with the mind in its quasi-physical state getting more of an assignment in the process than the soul because the mind needs to process infor-mation about the illness and its impact. But Dyer presents an intriguing idea for bringing the three aspects into balance, which is especially applicable in the time of a medical crisis: "See yourself as a soul with a body, rather than a body with a soul."[14] And he cautions that the mind does indeed help provide for the health of the body: "Thoughts heal the body, not the other way around."[15]

If you consider the flipside of Dyer's idea, you can see that dark thoughts and a wounded spirit will inhibit the body's abil-ity to heal. Dr. David Hamilton, writing for the World Council of Churches, noted that "unresolved guilt, anger, resentment, and meaninglessness are found to be the greatest suppressors

of the body's powerful, health-controlling immune system ... "
His idea was echoed in *The Healing Touch of Jesus*, by Rev. Dr.
Richard Lee: "Time doesn't heal all wounds. It really doesn't
heal any wounds ... Unhealed wounds are the unseen enemies
of the soul that provoke most of our suffering and failures."

Whole Person Approach

Uncomfortable as the members of the medical team may be
with the concept, there is a rapidly growing body of evidence
that demonstrates over and over again that a *whole person*
approach to treatment will produce better results than a *ratio-
nal/mechanical* approach, in which the physical symptoms are
treated in isolation. In its worst form, this idea of isolating
then treating a symptom limits the many additional forces
for healing that can be called upon in medical treatment. The
whole person approach is sometimes known as holistic, which
is another word that expresses the concept of synergy—that
the whole is greater than the sum of the parts. It makes sense
to treat symptoms of illnesses as part of a whole system and
not as just an isolated phenomenon within a body.

We've all known patients, or been patients ourselves, who
have experienced this isolated treatment. Think of people who
are being treated for ulcers, for example. I don't think there are
many physicians who would argue against the understanding
that an ulcer is a physical manifestation of stress, a nonphysical emotional/intellectual condition. But what does the doctor
do for patients with ulcers? Doctors usually treat them with
medication and a suggested change of diet. It's rare and wonderful for doctors to go beyond the physical symptoms and
talk to their patients about the source of the stress and how
they might reduce it through non-medical means that involve
the mind and spirit.

An ulcer patient could benefit as much from becoming part of a support group to learn problem-solving techniques or from learning prayer and meditation skills as from following a new diet plan. Yet the system of Western medicine in which most physicians are trained doesn't allow the doctor or other medical personnel to look outside the particular box that contains only physical causes and cures in order to bring all of the aspects of their patients into the recovery process.

Engaging the patient's fighting spirit is most often the way in which the larger aspect of a person is put to use in a medical treatment. As far as that goes, of course it's beneficial. But that effort seems to me to be largely an intellectual exercise, one in which patients more or less talk themselves into viewing their bodies as a battleground and into believing that they, assisting the medical team, will win the battle.

Four breast cancer patients—Susan Kuner, Carol Matzkin Orsborn, Linda Quigley, and Karen Leigh Stroup—argue persuasively against this model in their compelling book, *Speak the Language of Healing.* They advocate for changing the mind-set from a battleground to a spiritual journey, thus making room for the third aspect of the self to be engaged in the work of healing with both the mind and body. In order to achieve the positive effects of this three-part approach to the medical issue, the patients, those closest to them (their inner circle of caregivers), and the members of their medical team all need to share an understanding of what it means to engage the whole person, not just their bodies, in the treatment of the disease or injury.

My sister decided that the battleground metaphor really didn't work for her, so instead she used an image of a crystal-clear river gently flowing from the medical team's various therapies through her body, washing the cancerous cells away.

When I engage in intercessory prayer, I feel as if a beautiful blue light is flowing from God through me and then out to whomever I'm praying for. I don't believe it is a simple thing to "see" God's healing power, but as human beings with active imaginations, we certainly can find ways to visualize the holy help that we are seeking. It's another way of putting our non-physical aspects to work to support our physical well-being as both patients and caregivers.

Integrating Body, Mind, and Spirit

This integration process begins, as Dyer suggests, with honoring the body. Hating their bodies is an easy trap for patients to fall into when it is their bodies that are the source of suffering. It may be a mind-set that you have fallen into as well, blaming the patient's body for creating the medical crisis.

There is a real danger in placing blame for an illness or injury on the patient or the patient's body because it establishes a no-win scenario. This damaging thought goes something like this: patients, in some part of their minds, invited the illness or injury into their lives. They could, if they really wanted to, create a new, healthy consciousness for themselves and be *cured* of the current condition. When the condition persists, it's an indication that they and their bodies are in need of the illness or injury and won't let it go. In other words, it's their fault that they have their various conditions, and it's their fault if they don't get well.

The idea that we can knowingly create our own health reality is especially prevalent among people who follow strict health and exercise regimens and practitioners of what can loosely be described as New Age spirituality. In my opinion, the degree of control ascribed to the mind in this scenario is not possible. Our conscious mind doesn't have that kind of power because it is the smaller part of the self. We can help ourselves with its power, but we can't will a reality into being for ourselves.

Our consciousness has to share control with the far larger unconsciousness. We can get glimpses of this larger part of ourselves when we dream. It's a very deep and complex part of the self, and one that sometimes is at odds with the consciousness. For that reason, I don't believe it's possible to say we can consciously control the reality of our physical condition. We don't will ourselves to be millionaires, as much as we might want to have lots of money, and we don't will ourselves into serious illness or injury; nor do our conscious minds, on their own, have the ability to make a disease go away by creating a new healthy reality. The mind can, however, work in partnership with the body to assist in the healing process.

Dr. Andrew Weil, a Harvard-trained physician, is a best-selling author and leader in the field of what is called integrative medicine, medical practices that engage the mind and spirit along with the body in the healing process. He is the director of the program in integrative medicine at the University of Arizona, the first program to train physicians in this approach at a major American university. In *Sound Body, Sound Mind: Music for Healing,* he notes that the mind can both help and hinder in the healing process.

> In the many cases of healing I have studied, I often have seen that changes in consciousness precede or accompany physical healing, leading me to think that therapeutic efforts should be directed to the mind as well as to the body. It's not a matter of wishing oneself well or thinking positive thoughts; rather I think the problem is to keep the mind from interfering with the healing system.[16]

Dyer suggests you need to find a way to replace that attitude of blame, especially blame of the body, with one of respect, even awe for the body—the patient's as well as yours. That attitude of awe can shift the intellect—from which this body hate comes—into a positive mode, which produces those healing thoughts. But how does the shift occur?

The mind's role initially is to make sense out of what is happening to the body. It processes all the information about the symptoms and diagnosis in an attempt to understand what's happening. The emotions of anger and fear that Dr. Kubler-Ross charted are the byproduct of this intellectual effort to come to grips with a physical problem. The shift that Dyer writes about, in which the mind moves from blaming the body to honoring the body, is exactly what Dr. Kubler-Ross writes about in the process of coming to acceptance of the patient's condition. Often that shift is made through the help of people outside the circle of caregivers—therapists or counselors and support groups—who can be used by patients and caregivers alike to deal with these feelings in order to achieve acceptance.

When the patient and the caregiver are able to come to acceptance, then the body, mind, and spirit are aligned in working for the healing of the patient. To return to the analogy of the home, the three aspects of the self can be seen to be in balance and working in harmony when the system, or intellect, can support the home, or body, which allows doors to open for the free flow of the spirit in and around the home. When patients are able to honor their bodies and make use of healing thoughts, then there's room for the spirit too. Daily practices, such as prayer, meditation, and contemplation, round out the balance by bringing the spirit back into the treatment and healing process.

Choices to Consider

If the system that your loved one is being treated by isn't going to recognize or honor the connection of body, mind, and spirit, then together you will need to make some choices. You, as caregivers, along with your patients, need to decide how important the whole person approach is. If it makes sense to your patients that they incorporate this approach in their medical treatments, then a new treatment provider will need to be found who is willing to work in this larger arena. Ask friends, neighbors, family, and colleagues about their experiences. If you or your loved one belongs to a faith community, there may be a congregation member who can recommend an appropriate physician who would be willing to incorporate elements such as prayer into the treatment process. Some large churches even have referral lists of physicians who include spiritual elements in their medical practice.

Even when it's not possible to find a physician willing to utilize this integrated approach, it is always possible to find ways to include the whole person approach in your loved one's treatment. Techniques such as biofeedback, hypnosis, self-hypnosis, guided meditations, and creative visualizations all rely on the understanding that the mind can be a powerful tool in assisting the body to heal.

As Dr. Weil notes, the process is not to create a new healthy consciousness but to allow the mind to step aside in these deep states of relaxation and allow the body's healing mechanisms to work without interference. A woman friend who underwent a face-lift used a visualization of her tissue healing, which she is convinced helped her to recover more quickly than she otherwise would have. Interestingly, the visualization was provided by her plastic surgeon. Ask the medical team members if they have recommendations, and if they don't, look for outside sources to teach one or more of these healing methods to your loved one. Referral sources might include wellness centers, your health insurance provider, or your local hospital.

Like these mind exercises, issues of spirituality need to be raised with the doctor as well. Increasingly it is possible for patients to broach the subject to their doctors and involve them in prayer. It is becoming much more common for patients to pray with their doctors in a wide variety of circumstances—in the operating room just before surgery or in the examining room during a regular office visit.

Your loved one should feel free to ask to incorporate prayer or other essential spiritual practices into the work of the medical team. If the doctors, nurses, therapists, or technicians aren't comfortable with that, then your loved ones may want to find someone to treat them who will add that dimension to the treatment. When that's not possible, then you and your loved one will have to find a way to provide for the mind and spirit participation without the doctor. Pray when the doctor isn't around. Meditate or read sacred writings while you're spending time in the waiting room. Dr. Dossey points out that in general, physicians are trained to focus exclusively on the physical ills of their patients, and they may view offering their own spiritual beliefs as being outside the bounds of the proper practice of medicine. He suggests that caregivers and patients who want to involve the members of their medical team in practices such as prayer should simply ask for it rather than waiting for the doctor to offer it.

Voluntary integration of the three aspects of the self by the patient, caregiver, and medical team is crucial to the treatment and healing of the illness or injury. Understand the whole person concept and work to put it in place with your loved one.

Doing so will be one of the great gifts that you can provide to one another because it will benefit both of you by keeping you both whole.

Laughter as Medicine

One aspect of the whole person that can easily be neglected during a medical crisis is use of the patient's sense of humor. Emotions, a product of mind and spirit, definitely have physical effects. Tears of laughter or joy have a different chemical composition than tears of sorrow.

One of the best-known examples of using the mind and spirit to assist in the healing of the body occurred in 1964 when author Norman Cousins was diagnosed with a terminal crippling disease, ankylosing spondylitis, a degeneration of the joints, including the spine. Cousins's story, which he wrote about in *Anatomy of an Illness, as Perceived by the Patient,* was first published in 1979. Among its startling revelations was that laughter helped the author heal from this awful disease. It was a best seller for years and is still in print today.

Cousins didn't use laughter as a cure of his condition so much as he kept it in his daily regimen, purposefully seeking out opportunities to laugh in order to fully exercise what he calls his "affirmative emotions as a factor in enhancing body chemistry."[18] Cousins conceded that even after he came up with the idea, he had his doubts about its use. "It was easy enough to hope and love and have faith, but what about laughter? Nothing is less funny than being flat on your back with all the bones in your spine and joints hurting. A systematic program was indicated."[19] Cousins started methodically watching films of the *Candid Camera* television show and old Marx Brothers movies.

It worked. I made the joyous discovery that ten minutes of genuine belly laughter had an anesthetic effect and would give me at least two hours of pain-free sleep. When the pain-killing effect of the laughter wore off, we would switch on the motion-picture projector again.[20]

Cousins didn't come up with his strategy out of thin air. He was convinced that his illness was related to a chemical imbalance—a depression in his body's immune system—and his idea was to try to put the system back in balance with a whole person approach, which included engaging his mind and spirit along with his body. It's worth noting that part of his plan included not eating the usual hospital food, which was full of preservatives, sugars, and dyes. He wanted whole grain breads instead of white bread and fresh vegetables instead of canned. What we would describe now as a healthy diet in 1964 was unusual.

Cousins and his physician, Dr. William Hitzig, also carefully studied his body's response to his unusual treatment regimen and discovered that the laughter treatments produced an observable change in his body's chemistry.

We took sedimentation rate readings just before as well as several hours after the laughter episodes. Each time, there was a drop of at least five points. The drop by itself was not substantial, but it held and was cumulative. I was greatly elated by the discovery that there is a physiologic basis for the ancient theory that laughter is good medicine.[21]

Cousins's return to health was not solely due to laughter but was the result of his understanding of the link of the mind and spirit to the body and the need to incorporate those affirmative emotions of love, hope, faith, and laughter into his regimen of treatment and care. He accessed his sense of humor by taping into his childlike self. What could be more childish than a TV show that caught people doing silly things or Marx Brothers movies, which are probably among the silliest ever made? Laughter for all of us can come easily and deeply when we can rediscover the child within who still is delighted by silly things. As adults, we tend to forget that inner child and behave in a more serious, dignified way.

Certainly as the caregiver for an injured or ill person, you are taking the situation seriously. When my cousin William, who lived in France, was struggling with cancer and debilitating chemo treatments, his wife, Valerie, was struggling to keep the family of three boys functioning while she dealt with depression. He sent out an e-mail request to family and friends to keep them supplied with a steady stream of jokes and cartoons. "Laughing really lightens the day," he wrote.

Valerie told me after his death that they both benefited from the intentional inclusion of humor in their lives, as did their three sons. "We had so much to be serious about," she wrote to me. "It was good for all of us to find one small thing to laugh about each day."

Don't lose sight of Cousins's idea that laughter is a necessary component of affirmative thoughts that are going to help in the healing of the body. Wise people through the ages have understood this principle, which was summed up by Irish playwright Sean O'Casey when he observed that "Laughter is wine for the soul." Wayne Dyer notes that laughter is instinctive in human beings.

> The sounds of fun are the sounds that not only heal the body, but also heal the spirit... We all want to enliven our lives, to feel more connected to one another, to heal what ails... One of the simplest and most basic ways to achieve these lofty ideals is to spend more time just plain having fun and deliberately laughing out loud.[22]

Living the connection of the body to its mind and spirit is not always easy—we get out of balance even under the best of circumstances. You and your loved one are in an extremely stressful, difficult circumstance, in which it is easy to fall into the trap of focusing on the obvious physical nature of the medical problem. But I believe you both will be best served and that the blessings you need to seek out and hang on to will come when you can shift from the singular, mechanistic approach to one that integrates your minds and spirits in the medical journey. Yes, the holistic approach is for patients, but you, as caregivers, should not neglect it for yourselves. Make time for your spiritual practices every day; seek out the information about your loved one's condition so that you can learn all that you need to about caring for your patient.

As you move back and forth through the various emotional stages of the process, your goal and the goal of the patient ultimately is acceptance, which is truly the highest alignment of the mind and soul with the body. We are in an age that increasingly recognizes this concept, and so it is not impossible to find mainstream medical practitioners who can help you and your loved one to integrate this quest for wholeness in the medical procedures. As Dr. Dossey notes, it is "now possible to tell a new story, one that allows science and spirituality to stand side by side in a complementary way, neither trying to usurp or eliminate the other."[23]

PUTTING THE BASICS
TO WORK

LESSON EIGHT:
BEING WITH THE PATIENT

. . .

LESSON NINE:
EMOTIONAL/PSYCHOLOGICAL SUPPORT

. . .

LESSON TEN:

SELF-CARE FOR CAREGIVERS

LESSON FOUR:
THE DIAGNOSIS

September 16, 1999

So here I am, back in the same old soup. Dad told me today that his blood problems are something called aplastic anemia (later, we found out it was mylo dysplasia). And while there's lots that I don't know about the disease and his specific condition—and that I'm going to head for the Internet to start learning—I can feel myself slipping into the survival mode, circling the wagons, tearing sheets into strips for bandages, and counting ammo. This is too soon after MaryKay's death. I'm not ready to do this again. I know that his time is not infinite, and certainly that every day is a gift because of the lymphoma. But I had sort of pushed all of that understanding to the back of my head and ignored it. You can always hope it will go away while you're not looking. Once again, my choices need to center around how I deal with this—did I really learn anything from MK?

For me, bad news has always carried a quality that makes it stand out in stark relief from my other memories. Anyone who was living in the United States in 1941 could tell you exactly what they were doing when they heard about the bombing of Pearl Harbor. For my generation, those moments of clear recall swirl around the assassinations of John Kennedy, Martin Luther King, and Robert Kennedy. We all recall the moment of seeing the explosion of the Challenger Space Shuttle, and, of course, the destruction of the World Trade Center Twin Towers and the attack on the Pentagon.

Bad news on a personal level functions the same way. I can tell you in detail about the afternoon when I was sixteen that my mother told me she had breast cancer. It was a warm, spring day after school. Mom left a note asking me to meet her at the beauty parlor where she had a standing Friday afternoon appointment. I can still hear the loud background chatter of the other women who were sitting under the bonnet dryers and smell the combination of ammonia from permanent mixes, the shampoo, and the hair spray that perfumed the salon. And I can still remember how quietly Mom spoke when she told me that she and Dad wouldn't be leaving on their trip to Spain that weekend, that instead she'd be going to Pasadena on Monday to have surgery for a lump she'd found in her breast.

The same photographic quality of the moment applies to other instances of receiving medical bad news, such as the moment in a horse barn when I was told that my friend and trainer was in a coma with a brain injury or the moment at our office Christmas lunch in 1997 that my only sister told me in a very businesslike way that her breast cancer had recurred after the briefest half-year of remission. It is as if time stands still, and the sights, sounds, even smells of that moment create an indelible impression. *Oh no,* I thought each time. *This can't be happening.*

The patients—our loved ones who are the subject of the medical bad news—all report a similar response of remembered detail along with shock and denial as they wend their way through the medical process of determining their diagnosis. Rarely does the diagnosis come during an initial visit to the doctor. There's almost always a series of doctor visits and tests spread over a period of time before there's a diagnosis. Part of the delay is the natural response of patients to their own symptoms. No one wants to hear that kind of bad news, so we all have a tendency to frame the symptoms as surely being from some other cause, certainly benign.

Doctors and other medical professionals can seem to move with excruciating slowness while making a diagnosis of serious illness. They have to be as certain as possible that if they must give a patient bad news, it's accurate. The tests take time to schedule and time to complete. There are often a series of possibilities that need to be ruled out. The pain in Dad's shoulder and back might have been a strained muscle from an errant golf swing or perhaps some arthritis. A more serious set of possibilities were that it could have originated from some internal problem, perhaps something gone awry with his kidneys, liver, gall bladder, or other internal organs, all of which had to be checked out before the diagnosis of non-Hodgkin's lymphoma could be reached.

As awful as the reality of the diagnosis is, once it's given, knowing what they're facing is, in some ways, easier for patients to deal with than the dread of *all* of the possibilities. As in Dad's case, spinal problems, liver problems, and the whole list of potential medical horrors loomed much larger and looked far more overwhelming than the straightforward reality of the specific cancer diagnosis finally given. Free-floating possible diagnoses produce free-floating anxiety. Knowing specifically what the patient is up against, what its name is, and what its causes and treatments are helps provide focus that can reduce anxiety. This doesn't mean that a person who has been given a diagnosis of a life-threatening illness isn't going to be angry and fearful. The difference is that they know what they're angry and fearful about.

If it's a traumatic injury, a stroke, or a heart attack, the medical process begins with treatment rather than days of testing and analysis. However, that delay sometimes is useful in helping the patients and their family and friends come to grips with what's happening. In an injury or traumatic illness, there is no time to do that. The person is perfectly fine one instant and, within an hour or a day, hospitalized with the outcome in doubt. The mind doesn't want to accept it. We go back to the fact that our loved ones were perfectly fine just a day ago and keep asking ourselves how this awful circumstance could have happened so suddenly.

Yet the problem of receiving the bad news is the same in both circumstances. The fact of the matter is that everyone involved goes into a form of shock. My friend Cindy, the mother of three adult children, recalled thinking, *This can't be happening. I haven't finished my baby books yet,* when she was diagnosed with breast cancer. Like many patients who are given a diagnosis of a life-threatening disease, Cindy also recalled that the doctor was talking, but it was hard for her to actually comprehend the words that he was saying. She said it was almost as if he was speaking some language that sounded like English but actually was something else.

Dr. Nick Yaru, an orthopedic surgeon who was treated for prostate cancer, understands exactly how that shock feels: "*Telling* people they have cancer is difficult, one of the most difficult things a doctor has to do. *Being told* you have cancer is devastating. I remember going numb." That typical reaction of shock is one of the key reasons for adopting the team approach to medical appointments.

Information Gathering

As I mentioned in the preface, a universal and immediate response to the diagnosis is to gather information, which can be both good and bad. It's good when it enables patients to understand their disease or injury. This understanding helps them to make informed decisions about their course of treatment. But it's not beneficial when the information creates an overload in which they become paralyzed, unable to make a decision about treatment because of an overwhelming amount of factual data or because of conflicting information.

So how do you, as their supporter and caregiver, help them through the information maze? There are no easy answers, but a guideline for you—as a supporter—is to judge the value of information you find on the basis of how it may help your loved ones with the difficult decisions being faced. It's a fine line in determining what information is supportive, by offering some viable alternatives that they may not have yet contemplated, and what information is negative, because the alternatives offered aren't going to benefit your loved one.

Alternative therapies are a concern because you want your loved one to have all the options available, to offer the best outcome possible. But there are many well-intentioned people in our world who could derail your loved one's treatment by offering cures that aren't beneficial or that may even be damaging—and those are the well-intentioned people. There are also crackpots and outright frauds out there who will offer useless treatments for their own personal gain or sense of power.

Medical breakthroughs happen daily, and one may apply to your loved one. Gene therapies that could end diseases like cystic fibrosis and central nervous system disorders are not far off. Treatments that are common for cancer today were barely in the experimental stages a decade ago. Countless patients have enjoyed long and productive lives due to organ transplants, which are common now but were rarely performed twenty-five years ago.

But there is also a fair amount of bunk out there, which is not going to help your loved one. Be cautious! Look at the credentials of those who offer information. Ask yourself if the information has been clearly established in rigorous and repeatable scientific experiments involving hundreds of people. Or is it the idea or experience of one person alone? Be willing to let the medical experts have their say.

Mary Susan Herczog, who wrote in the *Los Angeles Times* in a series of articles on her experiences with breast cancer, offers a useful standard for judging the viability of information: if the proposed cure or treatment plan appears in an outlet that lacks the stamp of approval of established sources, then you have to ask yourself why it's outside the mainstream. Can it be that the wondrous cure being touted has been rejected as nonsense? Yes, some ideas that are initially rejected come back to being accepted by the scientific and medical establishment, but that acceptance comes only after rigorous testing of the idea. If the treatment is written up in a self-published book or appears on an infomercial or one-person Web site, you'll want to seriously question its use by your loved one.

Ms. Herczog explains her standard:

> [I received] letters from readers urging me to abandon chemotherapy because it does not cure breast cancer (news to my clinic and countless people), and to follow some natural method of healing they know about and have sometimes written books about—self-published because, they claim, the publishing industry is under pressure to keep this information from the public. (Oh, yeah, the publishing industry hates to put out books about cures for cancer.)[1]

However, the caution against some of the available information doesn't mean that all research is dangerous to your loved one. Far from it, if you have the skills to access Web sites of research centers and medical libraries, as did Laura Landro, a freelance journalist who was diagnosed with leukemia. Faced with the need of a bone marrow transplant to counter the progress of her disease, Ms. Landro says:

> [I] unearthed important data and medical papers that quickly educated me about my disease and the fast-evolving science of bone marrow transplants. What we found shook me up. But it also convinced me to withdraw from treatment at my local cancer center in New York and undergo a transplant at the Fred Hutchinson Cancer Center in Seattle, where our research strongly suggested my chances for long-term, disease-free survival were much better.[2]

My friend Cheryl created her own standard while searching out information on breast cancer after her diagnosis in February 2000. She went online, typed in the keyword *breast cancer*, and started checking out sites. She decided she wanted to benefit from the experience of other breast cancer patients, so she went for information on chat rooms and support groups. She connected to a group that was full of interesting, well-informed patients who had plenty of useful advice to offer her. "One of the best ways to tell good information from junk is to talk to long-term survivors and patients who've already been through their treatments," she said.

By seeking out advice from these former patients, Cheryl was able to make some informed choices, especially about the reconstruction of her breast. Given the controversy at the time over silicone implants, as opposed to saline implants, she was understandably concerned when the surgeon who was doing the reconstruction recommended a silicone implant. But she ultimately chose the silicone, not just because her physician recommended it but because of the numerous recommendations and positive experiences with silicone implants of the women in her online support group.

When our mother was treated for breast cancer in the 1960s, the only option following a mastectomy was use of a prosthesis, or false breast. Mom was always uncomfortable in sleeveless tops. Bathing suits were always a problem for her because she felt that the false breast, even though it was completely concealed, and the burns from radiation that scarred her shoulder and arm, made her the object of stares.

MaryKay had no intention of living her life that way. She told me she would have breast reconstruction using fatty tissue from her stomach. My job wasn't to help her sort out options but to be supportive of the option she had already chosen, which I was happy to be. On the day of her reconstruction surgery, I was dispatched to find a specific brand of lightweight girdle that would ease the pain while the site of the tissue removal on her stomach healed. It was a point of humor that we'd long ago given away girdles (in favor of panty hose), and here she was wearing one again.

Patient vs. Medical Consumer

Ms. Landro strongly suggests that you and the patient become medical consumers rather than passive recipients of treatment. Selma Schimmel, author of *Cancer Talk,* describes medical consumers as people who "clearly communicate their concerns, needs, and wishes; ask questions; understand treatment goals; and are able to talk with their doctors about whatever is on their minds."[3] Here are some ways that you can become a medical consumer:

- Start with the diagnosis itself, and assure yourself that the doctor has given you and your loved one all the information possible about the diagnosis and treatment that's being proposed. Ask *lots* of questions—is the diagnosis complete, or are there questions that still need to be answered; and if so, how does the doctor propose to get the answers? What is the outcome that's anticipated? How long is the treatment expected to last? What are the anticipated side effects? What is the anticipated cost, and how much is customarily covered by your loved one's insurance?

- Get the facts about the medical condition. If your loved one's physician gives you only a bare outline, ask for more detail or get additional information by phoning or e-mailing the local association related to the medical condition. If you have Internet access, go to one of the online bookstores and type in a keyword search with the name of your loved one's condition. You can either order off the resulting list or take it to your library to find the books. There will be several to choose from. The list under the words *heart attack,* for instance, produced more than a hundred titles. Ms. Landro recommends the National Library of Medicine (www.nlm.nih.gov) and the National Institutes of Health (NIH) at www.nih.gov. A relatively new site that holds a wealth of information for cancer patients is www.chemotherapy.com, and I have found www.webmd.com very useful as well.

- Don't be intimidated by technology. If you or your loved one don't have computer skills, you can probably find a friend or neighbor who can help. Your local library is a good place to start because it's likely to have a computer with free or low-cost Internet access and a librarian who can help you learn how to use it. Ms. Landro suggests that you stick to reputable sites that are connected to recognized treatment centers for the condition you're dealing with. University hospitals are excellent sites for information gathering.

- Don't be afraid of medical data. Ms. Landro says that while it may take some digesting—and the statistics can be a little frightening—they are worth the mining effort that goes into finding and understanding them. It's how she found out that there were three different ways to perform the procedure she needed. You can be a big help to your patient by finding out about the various treatments options and the health centers and hospitals where those treatments are offered.

- Don't assume your loved one's doctor knows everything. Your physician, unless he or she is *the* expert in the field, may not be using cutting-edge therapies or clinical trials that offer new hope where older treatments have not been effective. The NIH publishes clinical trials information. Dr. Rachel Remens, a medical doctor and therapist who works with patients with life-threatening illnesses, refers to a diagnosis as "an opinion and not a prediction."[4] When you and your loved one are reeling from the shock of the diagnosis, Dr. Remen's saying is a good one to hold in your minds.

- You and your patient can network with other patients and caregivers. Cheryl became very close to a few members of her online support group while she was being treated for breast cancer. They became such good friends and supporters of one another that three of them decided to get together on a regular basis, to continue to support one another. Ms. Landro notes: "You aren't alone. Don't hesitate to reach out; it may help save your life."

As a caregiver, you may be surprised how much you will need to know about your patient's condition. If you are going to support your loved ones, then you need to know about their diseases and the treatment options for them. Neither you nor your patients can be passive about accepting proposed medical treatments. You need to become active medical consumers.

Alternative, Complementary, and Integrative Medicines

One of the most obvious conflicts that arise in the information-gathering stage is between what I'll describe as traditional Western medicine and alternative therapies, especially the use of herbs in place of man-made medications. There are differing titles for these non-traditional medicines—alternative, complementary, or integrative. However you wish to name them, they are the treatments and practices that fall outside the traditional physician/hospital-based model.

Instances of the use of both systems of treatment can be found in the headlines regularly. In a study published in 2000, 69 percent of the cancer patients surveyed said they had used some form of complementary medicine, and 89 percent said they would like more information on these kinds of treatments. Eighty-four percent of surveyed parents of children being treated for cancer at Columbia University said they had their children using at least one alternative therapy in addition to the treatments given at the medical center. Cincinnati Children's Hospital uses up to eight nurses and licensed massage therapists who provide the young patients with healing touch, massage therapy, acupressure, and reflexology at no charge.[5] Surveys show that people with heart disease, arthritis, and other diseases are also interested in alternative therapies in addition to their traditional medical treatments.[6] Further developments in the integration of a wide range of therapies along with Western medical practices led *Time Magazine* in 2005 to create a grid of treatments for various types of pain, both chronic and short-term, and ranging from headache to neuropathy, which included behavior changes, mind-set changes, and physical therapies, along with pain medication. Clearly medicine is becoming increasingly inclusive of a whole body approach, which makes room for therapies outside of a strict treatment mode.

However, sometimes there is a conflict between the two systems. Television star and diet guru Suzanne Somers made headlines when she acknowledged that instead of taking a course of chemotherapy for her breast cancer she was using a mistletoe extract. Alternative medical practices, such as the use of herbal medicines, can be beneficial as an *addition* to Western medicine under certain, not all, circumstances. There are two fundamental issues involved:

- Herbs have chemical properties that will interact with other medications and with the condition of the patient's physiology. Just because it's an herb doesn't mean it won't have a chemical impact. Use of them, therefore, needs to be integrated by someone on the medical team who understands how the herbs will respond with the patient's particular circumstance.

- Herbal medicines are not subject to the same degree of quality control by agencies like the Food and Drug Administration as other drugs—even over-the-counter drugs. Consumers cannot be assured of the potency, safety, or cleanliness of herbal medicine to the same degree that they can trust the quality control in the more regulated, traditional medicines.

That said, it does not mean herbs are to be shunned. They can be helpful, particularly if your patient has a doctor or pharmacist who is knowledgeable and can help you use them in a way that assists or complements the other drugs being prescribed in the patient's treatment regimen.

At the recommendation of his oncologist, my dad used both acupuncture and Chinese herbal medicines to deal with the effects of the chemo he was being given for his blood disorder. For more than a year, he visited his acupuncturist/herbalist regularly and said he felt he was getting a great deal of relief from the side effects by following the dietary restrictions that the herbalist laid out for him. Unfortunately, as his condition began to deteriorate and the oncologist began using stronger medicines, the benefits of the alternative medicines disappeared, so Dad quit using them. He was not the kind of person who would normally have taken to alternative therapies, so I asked why he even gave it a try. "When you're as sick as I am, you'll try just about anything that can help," he said.

Dr. Barrie Cassileth, a researcher who runs the complementary care program at New York's Memorial Sloan-Kettering Cancer Center, says that herbs studied by medical professionals can be used as a complementary, not alternative, therapy.

If we know which ones work, and a patient comes in and says "I want to try herb X," we can say "Well, that may or may not be great but several others are helpful"...We have a tendency to think that just because something is natural, it's safe. But we have to be very clear on the fact that this is not always the case...some natural products like arsenic and hemlock, are outright poisons.[7]

Even Andrew Weil, a Harvard-trained physician who writes extensively on the use of so-called natural medicines as part of integrative and complementary medical practices, urges caution in the use of some of these therapies. He points out that standard medicine is best for dealing with traumas, crises, and life-threatening problems, though he advocates using dietary changes, relaxation methods, or herbal treatments for other, non-crisis medical conditions. If you or your loved one want to investigate alternative therapies, a good place to start is the Web site within the National Institutes of Health that provides information about alternative and complementary medicines.

Please be very wary of the so-called cures that don't come from recognized clinical sites. For shorthand, I'll call these bizarre treatments the *coffee enema cure* because they seem to regularly involve administration of some relatively common substance or a banned substance made from a common item.

Information about these extreme and extremely odd alternative treatments inevitably comes from a friend of a friend who has a cousin whose neighbor took this treatment and is completely cured of his or her illness. The only reason it's not on the market is a conspiracy involving the Food and Drug Administration (FDA) and the Big Drug Companies (BDCs). Or the person who invented/discovered it—and is making this cure available to anyone who's got the cash to pay for it—has been forced by the FDA and the BDCs to set up the clinic in Mexico, Haiti, or some other close-by, foreign country. Remember Ms. Herczog's warning about the self-published books about these *cures*. When you have no place else to go for treatment and hope, the coffee enema cure begins to make sense.

As I noted earlier, the Internet is a fool's gold mine for information about these kinds of treatments. Dr. Weil, who is an alternative medicine advocate, says, "There is a lot unproved in alternative medicine…I am not an uncritical friend of alternative medicine. There's a lot of junk out there—horrible, dangerous things you wouldn't believe."[8] Look closely at what is offered, and you'll probably find that the research that proves they are effective in curing the disease is questionable. By that, I mean it hasn't been conducted using generally accepted and rigorous scientific method, it hasn't been reviewed by the medical or scientific community (what is known as peer review), it hasn't been replicated by other researchers, and it hasn't been tested on a wide range of subjects.

Physician Larry Dossey, who wrote in *Healing Word: The Power of Prayer and the Practice of Medicine,* quotes from a study by Michael Lerner, PhD, who is president and founder of the Commonweal Cancer Help Program in California, an organization which is "devoted to service and research in health and human ecology."

> [Lerner has spent years studying alternative treatments for cancer and] has concluded that although there is plenty of anecdotal evidence that many such therapies improve the quality of life, he has not found any cure for cancer among the many unconventional methods he examined, and little scientific evidence that such methods extend life beyond what could be achieved with conventional treatments.[9]

Ms. Herczog, who used a combination of Western and Eastern medical practices in combating her breast cancer, is blunt about the dangers of a complete rejection of modern Western medicine:

> But I also think that those who would abandon Western medicine are foolish, if not downright stupid. Some who suggest this offer me anecdotes—someone they know who cured herself solely with herbs, someone else who died from chemotherapy. I offer an anecdote of my own, courtesy of my friend Robert, which I think shows everything you have to lose.

> "I have known three women who experienced breast cancer: my mother, my friend Elizabeth, and my sister-in-law, Pat," Robert said. "My mother and Elizabeth did chemo. Pat didn't want to lose her hair, so she did not. My mother and Elizabeth, many years later, are fine. You can guess what happened to Pat."[10]

Communication

Another immediate post-diagnosis issue will be communication. Who do you tell, and how much do you tell them? In her book, Dr. Kubler-Ross sets a high value on effective communication between patients, their family and friends on one side, and their medical team on the other. Censoring the flow of information among this group allows negative feelings, such as guilt, to control responses to the patient's medical circumstances, and that only keeps all involved in darkness. However, this process isn't quite as simple as it sounds.

The first problem that you're likely to encounter is its repetitive nature. Every person of significance in the patient's life, and yours, needs to be told what's happening. It can become an exhausting process. You will want to tell some people about the medical crisis in a face-to-face conversation. Depending on the nature of the illness or injury and the size of the group to be told, you may want to delegate the information sharing. When my neighbor was diagnosed with cancer, she asked me to let the rest of the neighborhood know, since she found it physically and emotionally exhausting to have to repeat her story so many times.

A second issue will be about the amount of information that's shared. At the same time there's a need for clear communication among the circle of intimates that surrounds the patient, there also is a need to limit the communication that goes to the wider world outside that circle. How much information is shared with whom can be a perplexing question. If the patient is a public figure, perhaps in politics, entertainment, or business, then there are factors outside the medical circumstances that must be taken into consideration: will the information create some wider response—a financial or political crisis, affect the chances of a sports team, or halt the making of a movie or concert tour? Who gets told about the condition and how much they are told needs to be weighed against the patient's need for privacy, as well as support.

One of the factors that limits the amount of information given out is the number of people who are to be told. If it's less than a dozen, then you and your loved ones can be as specific with the details of the circumstances as they are comfortable with sharing. When the numbers go up, then it's probably better to keep the details down to the bare minimum for this larger circle. One quick method to reach a lot of people with a minimum of effort is to use an e-mail broadcast. Obviously, this is *much* less personal than the phone call or face-to-face conversation, but it can save time and energy when getting the word out to a larger group.

There are also sharing Web sites, set up specifically for patients to be able to put out word of their diagnosis, treatment, and progress, which is another easy way to communicate with a large group. Rev. Davida Crabtree, the regional director of the United Church of Christ in Connecticut, used www.caringbridge.com to stay in touch with her many, many friends and associates as she was being treated for breast cancer. A similar site can be found at www.carepages.com. If you or your patient have a Facebook page, you can let your friends know that you'll be using it to update them on the patient's condition.

Especially in the shock phase of the serious, life-threatening diagnosis, the first inclination is to tell no one and just get through the process and back to normal as quickly as possible. When the illness is chronic or the injury disabling, then the issue of what to say and to whom cannot be avoided for long. I can offer no simple formula for figuring out this particular problem. The comfort level of your patients needs to be a primary guide—whom are they going to feel comfortable telling? Be cautious about severely limiting the flow of information when your patients are in active denial. A decision made at that point to not let word out about their condition and prognosis later on could mean they will not have the visits, cards, and other expressions of support that they'll want and need when they are no longer in denial.

Stonewalling can seem like an attractive choice on the basis that if you don't tell anyone, you don't have to deal with any potential negative reaction from outsiders. On the other hand, it can also cut off the flow of support that patients and their caregivers need and means that those opportunities for blessings go unexplored. I have two friends who both had the stonewalling experience with their mothers. The sad end to their stories is that the denial and stonewalling continued to the moment of death, robbing all concerned of the opportunity to experience the blessings of acceptance and healing of old wounds.

It's important to distinguish the communication that's required among the circle of intimates from the level that's required for the world outside that inner group. The outer world doesn't need to know all the details, the struggles, and the emotional hurdles that are being overcome. Sometimes that inner circle also gets left out of the communications loop for the best of reasons, but with *un*helpful results.

In my mother's initial treatment for cancer, she was cared for in a town more than an hour's drive from our home. My sister and I stayed home, sometimes by ourselves, while Dad stayed with Mom, who moved in with her sister to be nearer the hospital where she was being treated. As I mentioned earlier, we were teenagers. They decided to protect us from information they thought would upset us, so there were no opportunities to talk about how we felt about what was happening to our mother. Guilt, fear, and anger went unaddressed. They focused on her winning her battle, and that was what they felt we needed to know.

That same mind-set was back in place when her cancer returned seven years later. At that time, I had a young family, and we were living near my parents. But there were times when, rather than upset me, they wouldn't tell me Mom had been hospitalized. Unfortunately, when I found out she had been in the hospital for a few days and I hadn't been told, I was very upset, to put it mildly. Why had they shut me out?

In my experience, open communication between patients

and their inner circle, and involving the physicians whenever possible—even when information that's being communicated is distressing—is far better than a wall of silence, however well-intentioned that silence may be.

The contrast in sharing information when my mom was recovering from her initial bout of breast cancer and when my sister was recovering from her first round of treatments was marked. When MaryKay was diagnosed, the whole family talked about what was happening to her. Questions were encouraged, and that open approach worked well for all of us.

Knowing that key pieces of information are being withheld is very stressful. Inclusion of all close family members is the best long-term plan. For instance, MaryKay's then-teenage son chose not to participate in much of the communication with the medical team and family. I believe his unwillingness to participate—and his parents' unwillingness or inability to force him to participate—has left him emotionally scarred. He's in about the same place as MaryKay and I were when our parents intentionally excluded us from the communications loop.

Finally, I want to issue a caution in this call for full communication. While keeping the flow of communication among the medical teams and the patients' teams as open as possible, you may also want to limit questions from people outside the inner circle. That's where Web site-based communications can be so helpful. You simply post what you want people to know and refer them back to that site if they have more questions. Keep in mind, this suggestion covers people *outside of* the patient's inner circle.

The need to limit questions can happen when you reach a point that the patient or you have repeated the information about the medical condition, treatment, prognosis, and current status so often that it becomes burdensome to have to issue the same report over and over, no matter how well-intentioned the questioner is. I have one friend who doesn't ask questions, she interrogates. It's a quality that serves her well in her job, but I found it extremely stressful when she wanted to know about my sister. I realized I had begun avoiding her in order to escape her inevitable interrogation. I finally told her that I was uncomfortable answering questions and that I'd be happy to let her know about MK's condition, but that's all I was willing to say on the subject. MaryKay and other close family members also had similar situations, in which they learned to say to inquiries that were becoming too pressing, "That's really all I'm comfortable in saying." Note that if your patients are in denial about their condition, then they will want to call a halt to *any* questions. That's a different state from limiting questions that become too repetitious, detailed, or personal.

Shadow Experiences

I've noticed that when the word gets out about an individual's medical crisis, everyone who knows wants to be helpful. Family, friends, colleagues, and neighbors all jump in with good wishes, suggestions, and information. The intention is to be helpful and supportive, but that isn't always the outcome. There will be times when you will be confronted with what I call a shadow experience, a circumstance that, by its negativity, only deepens the darkness.

A woman who worked in our office building stopped me after MaryKay's initial diagnosis to ask how she was, what treatment she was undergoing, who her doctor was, etc. When I gave her the name of the doctor, I found myself in the midst of a shadow experience. This well-meaning woman launched into a twenty-minute tirade on how that doctor had utterly failed a close friend who'd died in agony, presumably as a direct result of the doctor's ineptitude or malevolence. I hadn't asked what she thought about the oncologist. What compelled her to share such a negative opinion? What did she think I was going to do with it—tell my sister she'd selected an incompetent physician? Rather than do that, I simply extracted myself from our conversation, said nothing to my sister, and avoided the woman as much as possible.

Another shadow experience you may encounter around the time of diagnosis will come from well-meaning people who offer up all sorts of information about treatments and claimed cures that are well outside the bounds of conventional medicine. I've talked a bit about the information you may uncover in "Information Gathering." This is slightly different. This is information given to you by well-meaning friends, neighbors, or colleagues.

Let me say here again that I do not mean to imply that *any treatment* not part of Western tradition, such as acupuncture or herbal medicines, should be regarded as useless. Some of these treatments—including naturopathy, homeopathy, healing touch therapies, and acupuncture, for instance—are effective as complements to the more traditional Western-style medical treatments.

What I'm referring to, in terms of shadow experiences, are *not* these widely used complementary medical practices but instead are the wacky ideas that are way, way out of the medical mainstream, treatments taken *instead of* conventional treatments, which some people will finally turn to in their desperation.

Sadly, I have had personal experience with these so-called cures. In neither case did they work. In fact, it's my belief that the patients lost precious time with family and friends by traveling long distances to receive these bogus treatments. In the case of one family member, I'm convinced that her death was hastened because of the damage done to her body by the particular cure she was taking.

In both cases, the person offering the cure was operating as a self-styled hero who was providing treatments that had—and would—cure patients suffering from a wide variety of illnesses. They always had very convenient reasons why they operated in a black market setting, reasons that would not stand up to close scrutiny. However, the patients were desperate, and in their desperation, they tended to turn a blind eye to the fake credentials and excuses and place all their hope in the miracle outcome. That's what makes the offer of this information a shadow experience as opposed to a blessing.

The Shadow Side of "Faith" Cures

A variation of the coffee enema treatment is the religion-based cure, such as laying on of hands, use of crystals, or faith healing. These kinds of cures cover the gambit of faiths—from fundamentalism of the world's religions to New Age practices. Let me be quite clear that I *do* believe there are ways in which faith, particularly when it's expressed through prayer, can be powerfully beneficial.

I am extremely wary of these so-called faith cures because I see that they carry a tremendously negative side that has the potential to plunge you and your loved one into deeper darkness. That's because this type of cure generally involves charismatic individuals who perform their ceremonies—be it laying on of hands or aligning crystals, whatever—on the patient. There's an important distinction in my mind between individuals using their special powers *on* a patient and having patients themselves and their circle of loved ones and medical team members invoke the spiritual dimension in the physical process of the treatment by joining *together* in prayer or other spiritual practices.

My strongest objection to the religion-based cure is the patient-responsibility context in which it's offered. That context usually runs along the lines that the patient is ill or injured due to some form of divine retribution, and if the patient has truly sought forgiveness, has sufficient faith, is pure enough of heart, or truly wants to be well, then the cure will work. On that basis, there's very little chance for the patient to have a successful outcome.

Karen Leigh Stroup put it in succinct focus in *Speak the Language of Healing:*

> There was only one problem with these lines of thought, both the scientific and religious: taken together they laid my cancer at the feet of God. Some of my more conservative Christian friends urged me to consider what I was being punished for. Some of my New Age friends told me there was a spiritual reason behind my cancer, and my task was to find it.[11]

God's plans don't always include curing our loved ones, however much we all want it. When the source of the medical crisis is perceived as some form of divine punishment, which puts the weight of the effectiveness of cure solely on the patient's behavior and faith—or lack of it—then the result can be that when the disease or condition is not cured, patients are left with a damaging sense of guilt and suspicion that the lack of a cure is somehow their fault.

In my opinion, these so-called faith cures are the same as coffee enema cures or negative information about the doctor or treatment plan. When confronted with these circumstances, you need to ask yourself what the outcome will be in the long run if your patients take a detour from their treatment path to explore these kinds of alternatives. In pursuing these avenues, are they going to reject or harmfully delay needed medical treatment? And worse perhaps than a delay in treatment, will the patient pursue something that leaves them feeling guilty and blaming themselves and their own unworthiness for their medical condition or for the lack of positive outcome from these so-called cures?

Asking questions about any proposed treatment, be it medical, alternative, or faith-based, is the best way to proceed. There are always legitimate questions that all patients have about the qualifications of their physician and the course of treatment being proposed. A second opinion is a helpful way to help a patient assess the value of both. In the case of a faith cure, is a second opinion being suggested by the practitioner, or is the offered cure based on complete acceptance of what this practitioner has to say?

In the meantime, what do you do when you're confronted by people who have these shadow suggestions to share? Reacting with hostility isn't useful. After all, they think they're doing you a favor by giving you the information. But you don't want to encourage them either. I have learned to say something like, "I appreciate your thoughtfulness. I know my loved one will want to consider all options." You're not saying yes, you're not saying no, and you've acknowledged the attempt to be supportive, however ill-conceived it may be. Of course, if they keep coming back, you may have to resort to blunt or even forceful rejection of what they're offering. You have to decide when the patient's best interest overrules the need to preserve the feelings of the person pushing the bad idea.

Another shadow experience you may encounter comes from the person who wants to minimize your loved one's condition. It happens in a couple of ways. One is from the person who, upon hearing the news about your loved one, will say something like, "Well, I know someone who has it so much worse than you ... " or "Well, you'll be fine. I just know it ... " It's my experience that these types of responses don't produce the expected cheery result because they deny the reality of the situation. If you're in any of the stages, except perhaps denial, then hearing this nonsense will probably elicit a response that only deepens the emotional state you're in. Karen Leigh Stroup, one of four breast cancer patients who wrote *Speak the Language of Healing*, notes that these kinds of responses to her illness don't make her feel better. "In fact, [I feel] just the opposite."[12]

Another aspect to this particular shadow experience is a kind of medical condition one-upsmanship, in which your loved one's condition is discounted because it's "only ... " "Well, you're lucky. Your mother *only* has kidney disease, and it can be treated. My mother has Alzheimer's, and it's incurable." In my experience with these situations, the best response is to simply smile and nod. Don't waste your breath or time trying to change the other person's point of view. If you are feeling particularly compassionate, you can spend a few moments commiserating with this person and then end the conversation.

It doesn't matter what the cause of the medical condition is. Whether it's the result of a disease, a gene, an accident, or a lifestyle choice, the medical crisis is real, and you and your loved one are going to be living with the stress, limitations, and difficult choices that it brings with it. The source—and the treatment—of the medical condition is irrelevant. It's still a time of darkness for patients and caregivers, regardless of what someone else may think about the circumstance.

Likewise, it's inappropriate for anyone to downplay the role you've taken on in terms of the time and energy you bring to your caregiving. "You're only dropping by a few hours a week." "How hard can your caregiving assignment be? Your mother is hundreds of miles away." You'll hear variations on this theme of downplaying the difficulty of the assignment you've taken on. Make no mistake about it; being a caregiver is a tough job, whether you are the only caregiver who's on duty twenty-four hours a day or whether you're the family member or friend who provides your care on a less frequent basis. It doesn't matter whether your loved one's condition is permanent or whether it's curable to some degree, or whether you're living in the same home or hundred of miles from your patient.

Caregiving is demanding and can sometimes feel like a thankless task. The stress it can induce can lead to dangerous levels of burnout. There are well-documented medical studies detailing the health dangers to caregivers from the work they do. Burnout is real, and it's very serious, physically and emotionally. Severe cases show up in the daily news when caregivers resort to murder, or murder and suicide, as the only way they could see to get out from under the tremendous burden they were carrying.

When you find yourself in the midst of one of these one-upsmanship shadow experiences, it may help you feel better to express your feelings. Setting the record straight is a perfectly appropriate response to these ill-conceived remarks. "I'm sorry to hear that your mother is suffering too. I feel that my mother's condition is also a very serious one, and I am very concerned about her." Or, "I understand how demanding it must be to be your mother's sole caregiver. I'm working hard too, taking care of my mother."

Second Opinions

Second opinions are very much a part of twenty-first century life, including the practice of medicine. Whether it's an expensive car repair, a bid to paint the living room, or a diagnosis and suggested course of treatment, we are used to hearing from more than one source. Most insurance companies require at least a second, if not a third, opinion before treatment is authorized, on the basis that more information may mean a better decision about the treatment. (For health insurance companies, this is the one that is most cost-effective.) Given the cost of treatment for any serious illness, it makes sense.

Writing in the *Los Angeles Times,* health writer Rosie Mestel noted:

> If you've got a serious or life-threatening condition, second opinions can also be critical. Has the full range of treatment options been offered? Is your doctor sufficiently specialized in your kind of case?
>
> If you or your doctor are uncomfortable with a recommended treatment, if your doctor can't figure out what's wrong with you, if you're not getting better or you can't get your questions answered—all can be reasons to seek second opinions.
>
> Remember: Many medical conditions can be treated in more than one way.[13]

But many times, if not required by their health insurance companies to get second opinions, patients will not do so. There are lots of reasons for this. The patients may feel a second opinion challenges their doctor's authority and that such a challenge, in the patients' minds, has the potential to damage the doctor-patient relationship. But there are other, compelling reasons, both conscious and unconscious, that keep people from going for a second opinion.

When my father was diagnosed with testicular cancer in 1991, when the cancer returned in 1997 as lymphoma, and when he subsequently developed severe anemia, I kept pushing him to get a second opinion after each diagnosis. He never said he wouldn't do it, but he never did it, usually putting me off with a desire to wait until this or that result was in before consulting another doctor. He'd always been big on second opinions. Don't just take one doctor's word for it, get another doctor to look at the evidence to see if they see the same thing, was his view. "Medicine is as much art as science," he used to say. "So why would you want to hear from just one physician?"

Yet, when it came to his own medical condition, there were *no* second opinions. A few weeks before his death, he was still defending his choice to not seek a second opinion. His rationale was that a much earlier visit with a prior doctor was the initial diagnosis (not so), and that visit therefore made his choice of the oncologist who was then treating him the missing second opinion. It was a statement that could not have stood up to even casual scrutiny. Clearly he was going to defend that series of decisions to not seek another opinion, so it would have been pointless to press the issue with him.

So why did Dad resist, along with countless other patients? I believe the reason has to do with denial. Second opinions are normally sought immediately after the initial diagnosis and before a course of treatment is started. Patients want to be sure that they are getting the right treatment for their disease or injury. This process is rational and almost scientific in its approach to testing the first doctor's hypothesis against that of a second or third doctor. It's an intellectual exercise. Unfortunately, this process is being undertaken by people who are in a state of shock, who are not necessarily at the most rational point in their lives. There's a high probability these patients may not want to have to hear the same shocking information again. It's like the character of the wicked witch, Evilina, from the musical *The Wiz,* when she sings the song, "Don't Bring Me No Bad News." It's not surprising then that they may want to avoid a second opinion.

Another reason patients might be reluctant to get a second opinion is that they don't want to get conflicting information. It's difficult enough to have Doctor A tell you that you've got a life-threatening disease and that you'll have to undergo treatments that will be extremely unpleasant, very expensive, and potentially life-altering. But it's far worse if you go for a second opinion and Doctor B tells you that Doctor A was correct about the disease but entirely off-base on the treatment. Now these patients are in a deeper dilemma. Who do they rely upon when they may be betting their life on the outcome of the treatment?

That was my father's experience with the lymphoma. The oncologist who made that diagnosis told him the course of treatment he'd been given six years earlier for his testicular cancer was not what he, the second doctor, would have recommended, leaving the impression that Dad's recurrence was in part to be blamed on inadequate medical care by the first physician. How do you weigh this kind of information? In my father's case, the first physician was on the staff of a nationally-recognized university cancer center, and the second doctor was the leading oncologist in our affluent community. I'm not surprised that patients are reluctant to expose themselves to this kind of medical second-guessing when it's their health and well-being, maybe even their life, at stake.

Generally, when patients like my dad aren't interested in

getting a second opinion, it's because they're focused on getting the treatment started, completed, and getting on with their lives. The lesson I learned from these encounters with Dad was to speak my piece—that *I'll* feel better if he gets the findings and recommendations of his physician confirmed by a second opinion—and then let go of the outcome. It was not an easy skill to learn, but it was *his* medical condition, not mine, so I needed to let him do it his way.

On the other side of that coin are patients who are in very deep denial who will get endless additional opinions in a vain search for a doctor who will tell them the diagnosis was incorrect. These patients won't quit trying and will continue to look for an opinion that supports them in their denial. While doing so, they may be rejecting treatment that will help them.

I think the same rule applies for family and friends in this multiple-opinion case as in the one-opinion case—speak your piece and then let it go. Berating your patients for seeking more opinions isn't going to cause them to come out of their denial and may just cause them to defend themselves more vigorously, thus prolonging the denial rather than ending it. However, if the behavior persists, you may want to encourage them to get professional counseling.

A Good Swallow of Life

In the immediate aftermath of the diagnosis, it's tough to find blessings in the shock and dismay of the reality that your loved one is facing. Yet light can be found in this encounter with a serious illness because it affords an opportunity for everyone involved, patient and caregiver alike, to live life in a new way. Rabbi Ben Kamin writes in his book, *The Path of the Soul,* that, "A breath of death yields a good swallow of life."[14] The gift of that good swallow of life that can be available to patients as well as their intimates is the great blessing in the darkness.

Dr. Kubler-Ross sees the confrontation of death within a loved one's potentially terminal illness as being a way for each of us to come to terms with our own deaths.

> I believe that we should make it a habit to think about death and dying occasionally, I hope before we encounter it in our own life. If we have not done so, the diagnosis of [a life-threatening disease or condition] in our family will brutally remind us of our own finality. It may be a blessing, therefore, to use the time of illness to think about death and dying in terms of ourselves, regardless of whether the patient will have to meet death, or get an extension of life.[15]

Mitch Albom, in his wonderful book *Tuesdays with Morrie,* had a revealing conversation about this very subject with his former professor, Morrie Schwartz, who was in the final stages of amyotrophic lateral sclerosis (ALS or Lou Gehrig's Disease):

> "Because," Morrie continued, "most of us all walk around as if we're sleepwalking. We really don't experience the world fully, because we're half-asleep, doing things we automatically think we have to do."
>
> "And facing death changes all that?"
>
> "Oh yes. You strip away all that stuff and you focus on the essentials. When you realize you are going to die, you see everything much differently."[16]

Nick Yaru, the orthopedic surgeon whom I mentioned earlier in this chapter, has had a personal experience that led to a great swallow of life on his part. In spite of his lengthy and extensive training, he concedes he had never really confronted mortality. "Physicians are trained to be perfect," he says. And in his case, that meant not accepting the medical failure that death represents, the antithesis of a cure wrought by his medical skills.

While struggling to balance his belief that "to cut is to cure" with the reality that "some patients don't get better," Nick had his own encounter with mortality. He was diagnosed with prostate cancer, the disease that had killed his own father. His response to the diagnosis was a depression so profound that he attempted suicide by jumping from a rocky cliff on the Southern California coast near his home. His life was spared, but his right arm and his vision were damaged. He didn't know if he would regain use of them sufficiently to return to surgery, and he still faced surgery and treatments for the cancer.

"It was like I had a form of amnesia," he recalled of the aftermath of his suicide attempt. "The first clear recollection I had about a week after prostate surgery was that God had intervened to save my life. He had saved me for a purpose I couldn't detect, but at that point, I gave up all control and turned my life over to God." Nick recovered from his depression, his injuries, and from his bout with cancer to return to his practice, but in a new way. By his own description, he is a far more compassionate physician now, understanding that there is far more to life than the "to cut is to cure" credo that had once been his way of being in the world.

"One gains perspective by experiencing physical, emotional, and spiritual challenges," he says.

That perspective is described by Karen Leigh Stroup:

One of the blessings of cancer is that it gave me fresh eyes for the beauty of the world. Healthy people walked right by a dogwood tree in full bloom while I stood entranced for a full five minutes ... There was a time when I was very sick and I could not do much more than sit up in bed and stare out my window and the world was reduced to what I could see between the buildings that framed mine. But it turned out there was action enough for several days ... People parked their cars on the side street and walked to the restaurant down the road, arm in arm ... I wanted to pat their hands, to comfort them, to tell them to enjoy this.[17]

What you and your loved one are facing are indeed uncertainties and challenges. But this offers also an opportunity to connect in a meaningful way to one another and in so doing to learn what is truly important in this gift we know as life. As Rabbi Kamin notes, "By embracing mortality, we gain humility, tolerance, harmony, and peace—and the power to transform our lives ... It teaches us patience, enlightens us with perspective, blesses us with wisdom."[18]

Sometimes the lessons are so brief and the blessings seem so small, you might miss them. One lesson I learned—the hard way—was to slow down to be with my loved one at her speed. I was hurrying to get to a visit with my mom. I was running into the house I'd grown up in, one that I knew every crack and crevice of. My mind, along with my body, was racing, thinking of all the things I needed to get done that day and calculating exactly how much time—to the minute—I could spend with Mom. And then I got the lesson: I tripped going up the front stairs and landed hard on my knees. It hurt! But that painful and humiliating moment forced me to stop, and it made me realize that I was going to be no good at all to my mother at the speed I was going. I needed that fall to remind me to slow myself down to be able to meet her where she was. At that time, she was barely able to get out of bed and get to the couch.

Banged-up knees were not exactly the "good swallow of life" that I was hoping for, but they were a blessing because they taught me how to come to my loved one where—and how—she was. It was a blessing of *being* and of releasing *doing*.

What You Can Do

BECOMING AN ACTIVE LISTENER

As a friend or family member, your most important assignment in the initial stage leading up to and immediately after the diagnosis is to make room for the communication that Dr. Kubler-Ross said was so necessary to doing the work of the five stages. That means sometimes you will be a listener and at other times you will share your thoughts and feelings with the patient.

Listening—really listening—is an important skill, especially in these first shocking, frightening days. Your loved ones may need to talk out their fears, their "Pollyanna" hopes, or even talk about anything *but* what is happening with them. They may want to rage against the unfairness of what is happening to them.

Active listening is a skill that requires some thought and maybe even preparation. Dr. Dorothy Siddall, a family practice physician at Kaiser-Permanente Medical Center in Santa Ana, California, leads workshops in active listening. Here are some of the elements she teaches:

1. *As a listener, you are fully present and listening.* That means you're not thinking about what you're going to say as soon as the other person stops talking. You're not making judgments; you're simply taking it in. You're there to listen, so don't interrupt with your own stuff.

2. *You are willing to be open and genuine.* This involves willingness to be as honest as your friend or loved one needs you to be. You have to be willing to hear some hard truths, and that's difficult to do. As supporters of someone who's ill or injured, we have our own work on the five stages to do. You may want to set a boundary while you are dealing with your own denial. That's

okay, but it could pose a problem if your patients are in their depression stage and want to talk about their losses. If your goal is to support your patients, you don't want to shut down their ability to share the things that are important to them. A balance between your needs and theirs has to be found. The extreme of this boundary-setting dilemma would be to approach your loved one to hear them out but to tell them you don't want to talk about their medical condition. In that instance, you're not engaging in active listening because you've excluded their needs in setting your own boundaries.

3. *Likewise, you are sensitive to their boundaries.* There will be places they don't want to go. For instance, if your loved ones are in denial, you may think it's important that they drop the denial of their Pollyanna approach and get down to the reality of their circumstances. But that's not your job. You need to let them lead. You're there to support them by listening, not by changing their behavior.

4. *You are willing to keep what they say in strictest confidence.* A key element of active listening is to provide a place of safety for your loved ones where they know they won't be risking exposure of what they say to *anyone* else and where their feelings will be honored.

5. *You are willing to let them go into those five stages, including the anger and depression.* This is a hyper-emotional time in the lives of patients and the people that they are closest to. Emotions will swing wildly, especially in the first days of the diagnosis process, so one of the gifts you can bring to your loved ones is the space to let them experience and express their emotions without being judged.

HOW TO "BATHE" PEOPLE

In her workshops, Dr. Siddall also presents a communication process designed to assist patients in getting in touch with their feelings and to enable the caregiver to provide empathetic support. It's a way of opening communication doors and exploring feelings, and it is appropriate in any of the five stages. Dr. Siddall uses the acronym of BATHE: B for what's bothering them, A for how it affects them, T for what troubles them most, H for how they are handling it, and E for giving them empathy.

Here's a summary of how she uses the system not only in her practice but in training physicians who are in residency training in family practice at Kaiser-Permanente.

- Start with a question of what's going on—what's bothering them. Obviously in the circumstance of the diagnosis or process of diagnosis of a serious illness, you know generally what's going on, but use this phase to find out which doctor has been seen, what test they've undergone, where they are in the process. It's a good idea to occasionally echo what they're saying as a way to ensure you're getting the details correctly. You might find yourself saying something like, "Oh, so you're waiting for the results of the blood test, and you can't see Dr. So-and-So until that's in hand."

- The affecting part might begin with a questions of, "How do you feel about what's going on?" This is a way to open your loved ones up to what they are feeling. Remember that the time around the diagnosis is when people can be in a state of shock and denial. It can be helpful to them to get back in touch with their emotions and to have someone to share it with. But also recall that anger is a stage that follows denial, so you may be hearing some of that. You have to be willing to let them have their range of emotions if you engage in this process.

- The T part, what's troubling them, may seem obvious, but be prepared for surprises. The quadriplegic may focus on the fact that he can't play golf any longer rather than on a host of medical complications he's facing. Asking this question can help patients to focus on what's really troubling them. What they have to say will help you to understand their feelings more clearly.

- "How are you handling that?" is the key question of the H part of the process. It allows you to support them by validating what they are doing to cope. It may be that in listening to them you realize they are overwhelmed and haven't begun to develop a plan or a means of dealing with what's happening to them. This is a place where you might be able to offer a few suggestions. For instance, if you have a person who's diagnosed with kidney disease and she is concerned about the dialysis treatments she'll be receiving, you might suggest she ask her doctor for literature, which will have helpful suggestions for dealing with the side effects. Or you might suggest a call to the local organization that supports people suffering from her disease.

- Empathy is very important. It is an understanding that is so intimate that you can comprehend the feelings and motives of your loved ones. You cannot *know* what they are going through unless you have suffered from a similar illness or injury. But you can be empathetic, and one of the best statements of empathy is, "This must be very difficult for you." Try to summarize the "affect," "trouble," and "handling" portions and give them a statement of support.

Finally, a good way to close this process is to tell your loved ones that you're glad they were able to talk to you about their circumstance. You'll both feel better—the patients because they've been listened to, and you because you will be in a better position to understand what they are going through and how it is impacting them.

Dr. Siddall closes her active listening training with a quote from George Eliot:

Oh, the comfort, the inexpressible comfort of feeling safe with a person; having neither to weigh thoughts nor measure words, but to pour them all out, just as they are, chaff and grain together, knowing that a faithful hand will take and sift them, keeping what is worth keeping, and then, with a breath of kindness, blow the rest away.

LESSON FIVE:
THE MEDICAL TEAM

February 5, 1998

MK had another blast of chemo today. Things got screwed up at the doctor's office. Somehow they thought she was getting the portacath put in today. (Is that how you spell it? It's a "port" to a vein they install surgically so they don't have to poke her with needles every time she gets chemo or has a blood test. It would have saved Mom a lot of pain and suffering if she'd had one.) One of the nurses, Kelly, was really crappy about it, but another one, Cheryl, knew she was showing up and what was supposed to happen. How hard can it be to keep an appointment straight? End result for MK was that she felt abused because of the way the staff—especially Kelly, the Queen of Crap—dealt with her. Whether they expected her or not, there has to be a better way of handling these kinds of surprises so that the patient doesn't end up feeling like a jerk. She doesn't need to waste energy on stuff like that.

A crisis in our lives is like having an elephant in the living room. You may do your best to deny you've got this problem by ignoring it, by walking around it, or even by decorating it with knickknacks as if you'd planned for it to be there all along. Regardless of how you treat it, the fact remains—there's an elephant in your living room, and something needs to be done to usher it outside or make peace with it before it starts crashing about and makes an elephant-size mess.

Your loved one's elephant is the diagnosis. The shock of discovery and then the denial phase don't change the fact that there's a substantial problem that must be dealt with. The first step is to figure out what to do with this great big beast that's lodged itself in your loved one's life and, by extension, yours. Even that process itself can break down into a series of smaller steps.

Gathering information is one way to begin. Learning as much as possible about the disease or condition and its treatment can then go on to support the process of getting a second, or even a third, opinion. All the information that's gathered finally will be put to use when the patient decides on a doctor and a treatment plan. However, before these choices are made, I think it's important to consider a philosophical issue. This regards the basic language of this medical process, and that, in turn, affects the way both doctor and patient understand what they are working to achieve.

Cure, Healing, and Treatment

Quite apart from the medical terminology related to your loved one's condition and treatment, there are the words that define the basic understanding of what everyone is working toward. Is it a cure, or is it healing? These are two very different concepts. The dictionary gives remarkably similar first definitions for both words—"to restore to health." Yet, if you read on, there are important conceptual differences between the two.

Cure is from a Latin root word for care and carries a connotation of someone providing a service or treatment that is aimed at getting rid of disease. Every day we hand over ourselves and our possessions to be cared for by someone else. Think in terms of your car. Your mechanic provides a service of treating it for ill-timed spark plugs or other function problems. Even getting a haircut can be seen as a cure for hair that's grown to an unruly state.

Healing differs in that it doesn't have the passive component of the treatment being given to the recipient by an outside agent. The underlying idea of healing is to involve patients—in all aspects of their lives—in the process of restoring wholeness. It's a word from Germanic and Old English sources and carries a connotation of producing wholeness by getting rid of "sin, anxiety, and the like."[1] The Old English root of healing relates to things that are holy and sacred.

Cure is outcome-oriented and is based on the idea that medicine will be successful in reversing the progress of a disease. To cure is a task taken on by someone other than the patient—the medical team—and its goal is a complete restoration of the patient's health. Healing has a more holistic connotation because it includes an emotional and spiritual context as well as a physical one. Because illness and injury involve loss of some physical aspect of ourselves, the goal of healing is to bring wholeness, which in the face of the physical loss is *also* acceptance of that loss.

Outcome and results are always important, but healing, as opposed to cure, can occur even when the disease ultimately takes the patient's life. Cure, then, is directed toward a restoration of physical health, putting patients back to where they were before the disease attacked them. Healing looks to restore the wholeness of the patient.

Treatment is what the medical team of physicians, nurses, pharmacists, technicians, and therapists provide to the patients in order to rid them of their disease, or to cure them. It encompasses the many ways in which they will work *on* the patient to halt or reverse the progress of the disease or overcome the effects of the injury. Healing, on the other hand, is the work that also involves the patient in integrating mind and spirit with the physical work provided on the body by the medical team. Healing includes the acceptance that Dr. Kubler-Ross writes about, a state that can occur when patients and their inner circle all accept the physical condition and whatever its outcome may be. That acceptance is not dependent on medical science supplying a complete return to physical normality. Cure is not always possible, yet healing always *is* possible.

The following is from *Speak the Language of Healing:*

> For me, treatment began with surgery, followed by six months of chemotherapy, then seven weeks of radiation.
>
> Was it a battle plan? Did it establish a line of defense? Would it be a fight to the finish?
>
> No.
>
> It was a rite of passage, moving into the next phase of a journey that would take me toward wholeness—minus a breast, but whole nevertheless.[2]

Dr. Dorothy Siddall, a busy family practice physician with the Kaiser-Permanente clinic in Santa Ana, California, notes that about 80 percent of what drives us to our doctors is not pure disease but rather a mixture of physical symptoms of illness plus the psycho-social manifestation associated with those symptoms. Dr. Siddall frequently sees stress-exacerbated conditions such as rashes, backaches, headaches, or digestive problems. The other 20 percent of her patients come in with pure physical illnesses and diseases, and of those, fewer than 10 percent are curable. "We can control, ameliorate, or prevent, but we cannot cure for the most part," she notes.

> [According to Dr. Siddall, healing] is a positive response to your illness. You can be healed even as you are dying of cancer. Healing is about transcendence, about discovering the important things about ourselves, each other, and our relationships. Healing, coming to wholeness, is simply integration of our bodies, minds and souls, and the healing of our relationships. It can occur on many levels.

Her view is shared by retired surgeon Bernie S. Siegel. "My role as a surgeon is to buy people time, during which they can heal themselves ... they can go on to true healing, not merely a reversal of one particular disease."[3]

Physicians don't always share the distinction between cure and healing with Dr. Siddall and Dr. Siegel. Most physicians rely on their extensive training to devise a treatment plan, and in their minds, that plan has a positive outcome. As Dr. Nick Yaru noted, the problem is that patients don't always get well, which poses some philosophical problems for the medical team. One way in which some doctors resolve that particular philosophical problem is to blame the patient for not being cured. The result is to literally abandon the patient—if you won't get well and you don't want to keep trying new treatments, go find another doctor.

One case, which involved the twin sister of Rev. David Beadles, a recently retired hospice chaplain, was obviously an extreme. Moments after Rev. Beadles's sister declined further treatment from her oncologist in order to live out her remaining days with some quality of life, the hospital informed the siblings that she would be discharged *immediately,* since she was no longer under the care of that physician. The unspoken message was: "You won't be cured the way we want to cure you, so get out."

There are countless instances in which the tension over the issue of cure versus healing arises between physicians and their patients. Talk about this issue with the medical team. By starting with an understanding of the essential difference between these two concepts, both sides—the patient and the medical team—can alleviate some problems that might develop later in the process.

The Medical Team and Its "Captain"

How did your loved one get into the medical system? Was it through a primary care physician, who diagnosed an illness that required a specialist? Was it through routine screening or tests that showed an anomaly? Perhaps there was an accident leading to an injury, so your loved ones started their medical journey in an emergency room. The system that provides medical care in the United States is complex and can seem confusing and overwhelming, especially in those first shock-filled days.

With serious illnesses or injuries, medical care is provided by a whole team of professionals, and it's extremely important for you and your loved one to know who's on the medical team and who the captain is. You want to know not only the names, faces, phone numbers, and addresses (e-mail too, if you can use it) of the medical team members, but you'll want to have an understanding of their operating style—who's brusque and businesslike, who's vague in giving out details, which offices run on time, which always run an hour late, which doctors will take the time to talk, and which will limit the time they spend with patients. That knowledge can assist you in building and maintaining a good working relationship with all the members of the medical team.

When my sister first discovered a lump in her breast, she went to her gynecologist, who referred her to a radiologist to have a mammogram taken in the effort to determine if the lump was a benign cyst or a cancerous tumor. In the months that followed, MaryKay also had a surgeon who performed the mastectomy, an oncologist who was responsible for her chemotherapy, an oncological radiologist who provided radiation therapy, and a reconstructive surgeon who rebuilt her breast when the treatments were over. Each of those physicians had a full staff to assist them—nurses, nurse practitioners, vocational nurses, and office support staff.

With an array of medical expertise like that, you'll want to know which doctor is in charge of coordinating your loved one's care—which physician is the central information-gathering point, the one who specifically knows what the others are doing, what drugs they're prescribing, and when the treatments are scheduled in relationship to each other. In her case, it was her oncologist. If your loved ones don't know or if none of the medical personnel treating them has become captain of their medical team, then you need to figure out who that will be and make sure the whole team knows which physician is doing the coordinating so they can exchange information.

You also need to be clear that it's a one-captain team. Keeping life simple is important in this process, and nothing will create worse confusion than having two or more physicians assuming that they're in charge. Medical care is complex. You don't need to have it confused further by having doctors who are issuing contradictory orders regarding treatment.

Within the medical team itself, each of the physicians will have their own staff, and you also need to know who they are and what their various responsibilities are. The appointment clerk isn't going to tell you what laxative to buy for the constipation that your loved ones may be suffering from because of the drugs they're taking. Likewise, the nurse, nurse practitioner, or other professional in the office isn't going to book your loved one's appointments. Which member of the staff is the person to talk to about your loved one's medical condition when you can't talk directly to the doctor? Most medical offices have one person who handles calls from patients, evaluates them, and makes the decision whether to pass them on to the doctor. Get to know not only who those people are but get to *know* them—it will make your conversations more effective.

In addition to the physicians and their staff, you will develop a working relationship with a pharmacy and, if you're fortunate, with an individual pharmacist. It will be your pharmacist who gives advice on how to take the medicine—with food or not, eliminate dairy products while taking a certain drug, don't go into the sun, etc. And it can be the pharmacist who will note a clash between drugs prescribed by different doctors on the medical team. Get to know your pharmacist, or if you use a supermarket pharmacy or large chain drug store, get to know as many of the staff pharmacists as possible. They can be valuable in assisting with information about the drugs your loved one is taking.

Therapists and technicians who deal in the physical recovery of your loved one are also important members of the team. These may include physical therapists, occupational therapists, speech therapists, or music therapists, to name a few. I include in this category any of the professionals who actually provide a treatment to the patient. For instance, dialysis technicians are key team members to kidney patients. When the illness or injury requires a change of eating habits, a dietitian can be an important member of the team. Very often, the services of these technicians and therapists are prescribed by the attending physician—the team captain—so they are automatically part of the team and know who the captain is. However, don't assume that to be the case. Make sure their reports on your patient's progress get back to the lead physician and that the treatment plans involving other team members are conveyed to these therapists and technicians.

There will be lab people who do the tests ordered by the various doctors. Their work is obviously important, although you may not have the opportunity to work with them on a regular basis. That's because the lab work may be sporadic and occur only in relation to surgery or other modes of treatment. However, when your loved one needs regular lab-administered tests, then you will get to know who the techs are and should consider them part of your loved one's medical team.

Some of the members of the medical team are going to be easy to work with, always pleasant and concerned about your loved one and you. Others are going to present problematic behavior. My eighty-six-year-old neighbor encountered a lab tech who apparently decided that she was senile because of her age, and therefore he could ignore everything she said—including her insistence that the position in which he placed her for a scan was excruciatingly painful due to a rotator cuff injury. Or the woman who set up appointments in another lab who felt compelled to lecture me about her procedures because MaryKay's doctor had not contacted her in advance when I called for an appointment for my sister.

Occasionally, I find it entertaining to be relentlessly cheery in response to rude behavior. That's because I have a feeling that sometimes people are hard to get along with in the hope—conscious or unconscious—that their behavior will elicit equally rude behavior, and they will then feel justified in their unpleasant tactics. In that case, someone who is relentlessly sweet and kind is probably harder for them to cope with than someone who returns rudeness for rudeness. Obviously, you have the option of being as rude and unpleasant to them as they are to you. Or you can report their behavior to their superior—something my neighbor did.

The Patient's Team

Just as there is a medical team, I strongly recommend that there be a team for the patient. Facing the array of medical team members can be daunting, and it can only benefit your loved ones if they have their own team backing them up in this strange new world they've been forced into. This doesn't have to be a big team—just one other person can constitute a team for the patient within the medical realm. I believe that it's psychologically important for patients to have someone literally at their side when they are dealing with the medical team. Anyone, even a physician who has become a patient like Nick Yaru, can become intimidated by the medical process they are undergoing. There's a lot of comfort in having someone along who is on their side.

If there is no other suggestion that you take from this book, take this one idea: get your loved ones to agree that they will *always* have another person with them at *all* meetings with members of the medical team. Obviously, since these meetings will often include medical examinations, this second person needs to be someone who is close, who is trusted, and with whom the patient is completely comfortable. This is a most intimate assignment because of its physical nature. Your loved one's body will be examined and discussed, so the person who shares this experience must be someone the patient absolutely trusts. A spouse, a life partner, a parent, an adult child, a sibling, and a lifelong friend are all reasonable choices.

When it's not possible to have a second person along for the appointments, another good choice is to bring along a tape recorder, either a single cassette type or a mini recorder. That way the patient can play back the conversation with the doctor after the visit to get the details that may have been missed in the original conversation.

Selma Schimmel, a former cancer patient and founder of the radio talk show *The Group Room*, calls this member of the patient's team an advocate. She notes that sometimes, when the doctor's diagnosis or treatment plan needs to be questioned, the patient may be reluctant to do so, and so the task falls to the advocate. It's not always an easy job, but it's one that's vitally important to the patient. And because this is such an important task, it's equally important that there be only one person who takes it on.

Just as there can only be one captain on the medical team, so there should only be one advocate on the patient's team. Too many voices advocating for the patient are merely going to cause stress-inducing confusion and frustration. Patients and their loved ones have enough stress to deal with, so keeping stress to a minimum, where possible, has got to be a high priority.

My sister's advocate was her husband, Chuck. Due to his job, there were a few times when he couldn't go with her to appointments. So I became his stand-in. In those instances, I didn't become a substitute advocate so much as I just filled in for the function of doctor-visit scribe, the second set of eyes and ears for the visit. I left the advocacy—the staying on top of treatment plans and options—to Chuck and MaryKay. Later, when Ané de Nio came to stay with my sister, she assumed the role of sub-advocate, sharing her observations and questions with Chuck and MaryKay. It wasn't always easy because Chuck and Ané have two very different life views. They had some strong differences of opinion a couple of times. But what kept the system functional was their love of MaryKay and underlying desire to support her in her treatment.

Medical Meetings

There are a couple of very good reasons why your loved one needs an advocate in these medical meetings. First, especially during the initial diagnosis phase, there is just an overwhelming amount of information that's being given to the patient, more than anyone can realistically hope to take in. When my father was going through the tests that ultimately led to his diagnosis of non-Hodgkin's lymphoma, my stepmother, Claudette, began going to his appointments with him, armed with a pen and a stenographer's notebook. She made it a continuing habit to go with him and to take detailed notes throughout his illness. Sometimes it was amazing to hear the disparity between my dad's explanation of what the doctor said and what her notes indicated. He got most, but not all, of what she recorded of what the doctor had to say about his condition or the treatment plan. At some appointments, he picked up on more of the information than at others.

Another good reason for having that second set of eyes and ears in a medical appointment is because of the shock factor—both physical and psychological. When people are put into the shock-inducing circumstance of being told they have a life-threatening disease, they don't always hear clearly what's said. The people in my life who've been diagnosed with serious illnesses all report that after hearing the initial bad news, they struggled in their shock to hear the rest of what the doctor was telling them. Cyndy, a member of my church, said she remembers asking the doctor to tell her again what he'd just said because she literally could not comprehend the words.

As rational beings, we assume that we'd want to be fully alert and take in every bit of information that's being offered about our medical situation. The problem is that our bodies are wired for fight or flight when our lives are threatened, and a medical diagnosis of serious illness can produce that same adrenaline response that shuts down our peripheral systems in order for us to take on the adversary or run from it. This applies to you, as the team member in the medical appointment, as well as your patient. Just because you and your loved one are safely seated in an examining room doesn't mean that your bodies aren't going to respond to the threat. The peripheral systems will still shut down, which means that taking in a lot of information may not be physically possible.

There is also the response to our own pending mortality, which operates at a cellular level in living organisms. M. Scott Peck, MD, the psychiatrist-turned bestselling author, explains the power of this force in his book, *Denial of the Soul: Spiritual and Medical Perspectives on Euthanasia and Mortality*. He describes Freud's understanding of Eros, or the life force, and notes that in describing this life force, Freud "meant everything involved in the urge to live and grow ... This force is not merely psychological; it is embedded in every cell of our bodies. That is why it is not easy to die; each of our cells shrieks out against the necessity."[7] It makes sense that when shocking medical news is presented, our psychological response would be to filter out that life-threatening information. The ears may be picking up what is said, but the brain may be trying very hard to *not* process those sounds into information that indicates our life is at risk, denial at its most elementary level.

Finally, it's helpful to have this second person in the meetings with doctors to ask for—insist, if necessary—time in which the patient can ask questions. In most medical appointments, particularly diagnostic ones, it's the doctor who asks the questions, not the patient. Physicians who work with patients requiring long-term or intensive care may be more accustomed to having the patient ask questions, but don't assume that such will be the case with your loved one's doctor. As the patient's team member, you can provide a valuable service by merely getting the doctor to take some time to answer your loved one's questions.

Advocate/Scribe/Records Keeper

Your job as the patient's advocate is to be the scribe and, if necessary, keeper of medical records. You may be amazed to discover how easily a patient's charts, treatment records, diagnostic test results, X-rays, and the like get mislaid. Copy and maintain a file of as many of these as possible. The patient's medical records, while they are *about* the patient, actually are the proprietary property of the physician, the group medical practice, or the clinic that originates them. However, most doctors will, sometimes for a fee, let patients make a copy of the records that they can keep for themselves. That's because this information frequently has to be shared among the members of the medical team. It's in your loved ones' best interest to have a set of their own records under their own control. The one area where you may not be able to hang on to copies of records are films—things like X-rays, CAT scans, and MRIs, which are single-copy items. The medical team will want to hold on to the originals, but you can usually obtain copies of them on a CD.

You will be surprised to discover how much time is wasted when these kinds of records are misplaced, which they inevitably will be at some point in the process. The longer and more complex the treatment, the more likely records will go missing. Of course, the process of acquiring copies of a patient's medical records has been complicated by recent patient privacy laws. Because of medical information privacy laws, only the patient can request and receive copies of his or her medical records.

You will also be recording the patient's questions as you go to these appointments. There will be the drive to the office or clinic then the inevitable wait for the doctor, therapist, or technician. While you and your loved one are waiting and chatting, think of questions and *write them down*. You may want to expand this process slightly and play reporter. Before the appointment, prompt your loved ones to recall all their questions so you can get them written down to take along. In going to my sister's appointments, I found that often my most important function was to remind her of the questions she'd planned to ask her doctor. Doctors have their own agenda, and in following it, patients can sometimes get off the track of the information they need to have. Prompting questions is a great service that you can provide your loved ones.

Obviously, it's also very important in this scribe job to write down what the doctor has to say. This includes everything from discussions of side effects and progress, to changes in treatment plans, to reminders about therapies and beneficial or dangerous behaviors, to recommendations regarding medication. The more complex the treatment, the more essential it is for the scribe to help the patient to keep track of what he or she is to do or to not do. Those notes, combined with outside information that you and the patient have gathered, will become the basis of whatever advocacy needs to take place. In recording these notes, it's also a good idea to repeat them back to the doctor to ensure that you've written them down correctly. Yes, it will make the appointment last longer, but it's absolutely vital to have correct information, so it's worth the additional time it takes.

Dad was in the hospital for the third time in eight months when we called a family meeting with him and his oncologist. One of our family members is a physician's assistant, and she came along to help with the translation of information between the attending doctor and the rest of us. We wanted to know what to expect, since it appeared there had been a significant change in Dad's situation. The doctor did a great job of summarizing the five-year progress of Dad's disease and its treatment. I took notes, my stepmom took notes, and our family member PA listened intently and asked what I thought were good questions. The meeting ended with the doctor asking Dad what he wanted to do and Dad declaring that he wanted to keep fighting.

"I'm not ready to give up or give in yet," he said, according to my notes. As a former journalist, I think I can do a fair job of recording a meeting like that.

We had a very unpleasant surprise a few days later after Dad got out of the hospital and returned to the doctor's office for his regular treatments. The staff, after much embarrassed confusion, had to tell Dad that he was no longer scheduled for any additional treatments because the doctor had told them that he'd given Dad a terminal diagnosis.

The emotional pain and confusion that resulted from that very significant miscommunication left all of us feeling as if we were a little crazy, until we went back to our notes and consulted with our family member, the PA. None of us had heard anything remotely resembling a terminal diagnosis. The doctor may have thought he'd spoken it, but he had not. You can see why you want to keep track of what's said—or not said—in these meetings. The work you and your loved one have to do is difficult enough without you missing a hugely important piece of information, whether that gap actually occurs in fact or in the minds of the participants.

This significant communication breakdown occurred in the last few days of Dad's life, so the family chose not to revisit it with the doctor. Had the circumstances been different, I believe that we would have made an appointment and, as a group, had a meeting with the oncologist to discuss communications.

Maintaining a balance between the family's concerns and the doctor's expertise is a matter of being clear about what the family perceives the problem to be. It's the old standard—speak your truth without shame or blame. Any human being is going to be defensive if confronted by a roomful of people with a complaint.

Here's an outline of how we might have voiced our concerns (being careful not to label it as a complaint): "We heard you say this but not that. We're confused as to how we could have missed such a significant piece of information. We want to clarify where we are in our loved one's (diagnosis, treatment, prognosis) right now, and we'd like to figure out a way to keep our collective communication more clear in the future."

As you can see from this experience of ours, another reason to have the patient and a second person in on the appointments is for the two of you to compare notes afterward. As I noted earlier, Dad and Claudette usually came away from his appointments with differences in their understanding of what the doctor said. These differences were not always substantial; sometimes they were quite minor, and usually it was

Claudette's notes that were relied upon for clarification. But where there's a question of substance, such as we experienced, it needs to be clarified with a follow-up phone call to the nurse or sometimes the doctor.

When your loved one's health, maybe even life, is at stake, it is important to be sure that everyone involved is clear about what is done and said by the medical team. During this post-appointment debriefing, you and your loved one will probably come up with a new question or two to put on the list for the next appointment.

One final thought about the patient's team: you—as a supporter, caregiver, or advocate—are a team member. The patients, your loved ones, are the captains of their team. It is their medical condition. They call the plays. You can assist in gathering information, advocating with the medical team on their behalf, and suggesting ideas. You can inquire about decisions they've reached, but you cannot attack those decisions by questioning their validity. Your advocacy has to reflect the patients' wants and needs, not yours. You are not on the team to be in charge. You are there to support your patients. Remember, it's their body, so it's their choice.

Communicating with the Medical Team

In my opinion, it's not possible to have too much communication between the patient's team and the medical team. As you will discover when you start gathering information, there's a lot to know about whatever your loved one's medical circumstance is. A good motto for you and your loved one to adopt is: "If you don't know, ask." In the case of your loved one's illness or injury, the stakes are as high as they can be, and, as a result, both of you should feel free to ask the medical team members about any and all of it.

Urge your loved ones to keep their own notebook and pen handy, twenty-four hours a day, to write down questions as they occur to them and to note reactions to drugs and treatments—when do the side effects or symptoms get worse, when do they seem to be lessening? You may want to do the same thing. The simple truth is that we cannot remember all the questions, thoughts, or ideas that occur to us. Unless these thoughts are promptly written down, they will be forgotten. Remember that loss of concentration and short-term memory can be a side effect of surgery and chemotherapy. Nothing is more frustrating than to have some precious time with a key member of the medical team and for the patient or you to not be able to remember what to ask.

A good reason to keep pen and paper handy is for patients to keep a record of their symptoms—what makes them worse, when they occur, and when they wane. This information will be valuable in assisting the medical team in the selection of treatment plans, therapies, and drugs.

Another reason for the notebook is to track conflicting information coming from different members of the medical team. This is a good reason to be sure both the patient and advocate know who's in charge of the medical team, because these conflicts of information will arise from time to time. The more people involved in administering the treatment, the more likely it is that these disparities will occur. Don't let it alarm you. Expect it but have a means of resolving the problem. Note the conflicting information and present it to the lead physician, then make sure that whatever the problem is has been resolved. Don't assume the doctor will handle it. Be sure you know what the plan for resolving the problem is then follow up with all concerned to ensure that resolution has taken place.

Self-managed Care

One reason for a high level of communication between doctors and patient is what can be best described as self-managed care. This is about your loved ones being informed, proactive consumers of the health care services they are receiving. It's the reason for research and seeking a second opinion to ensure that the treatment being offered is the right one for the medical condition that involves your loved one. Once treatment begins, it shouldn't mean that information gathering ends. When your loved ones have found information about their condition from an outside source, they should feel free to take it to the appropriate member of their medical team to find out if, or how, it may apply to them.

Recall that Laura Landro, writing in the *Los Angeles Times,* advocates that patients follow her example of self-managed care in continuing to research their disease and its recommended treatments.

> While the Internet has revolutionized patients' access to information, managed care has made it more difficult for some to seek outside medical opinions or to travel to distant treatment centers where they might have a better chance of a cure. That has made it all the more important for patients, armed with knowledge, to manage their own care. And remember, sometimes a doctor can be your ally when dealing with your health plan, fighting for you and supporting your quest for the best possible care.[4]

Ms. Landro also urges patients and caregivers alike to become advocates, to talk to the members of their medical team about questions that arise from their information-gathering. She calls it talking back to your doctor and urges that this skill be learned in an assertive but non-aggressive way.

Many doctors are uneasy about this new era of the self-educated patient; they see you coming with reams of printouts from the Internet, and they groan. But some doctors appreciate a patient who cares enough to do his or her homework and asks intelligent questions. If your doctor seems nonresponsive, seriously consider switching to a doctor you are more comfortable with.[5]

One of the reasons for you and your loved one to be informed medical consumers is the simple fact that not all physicians are attentive during office visits. This known gap in physician communication skill has led to a new test that has become part of the licensing procedure for doctors who have completed their training. "Qualities such as listening carefully, noticing body language, and showing empathy may sound like fluff. But there's evidence that patients who feel rapport with a doctor are more likely to comply with orders and do better medically," says Donald Melnick, president of the National Board of Medical Examiners, cosponsors of the medical licensing exam. The new test will judge students on a variety of patient-oriented abilities, including ability to elicit information on symptoms, to create rapport and trust, and to communicate clearly.[6]

And don't be afraid to make rapport with the physician as important in the selection process as medical expertise:

> After being diagnosed with breast cancer, Mira Haimovich looked for practitioners who acted as if they cared. Her oncologist, she says, inquired about her feelings. Her radiologist, she says, "would always ask me how I'm doing, what's going on. He never seemed to be in a hurry." Her standards applied to alternative practitioners as well. Haimovich dumped one acupuncturist because "I didn't feel I was getting that nurturing."[7]

Tests, Treatments, and Procedures

Perfecting your communication skills with the members of the medical team is also important when tests, therapies, and treatments are being ordered by the doctor. Patients and their team members need to be very clear about what's to be done and what the expected outcome will be. The patients' team members may even want to be with them while they are being prepped for a treatment or procedure.

Medical personnel who provide the treatment ask a lot of questions, and if your loved ones aren't clearheaded because of medication or the condition itself, then they aren't going to be able to answer these fundamental questions—what procedure are you having done today being one of the basic questions asked. If you think it's a good idea for you to be present while your loved one is being prepared, then clear it with the treatment facility or medical team captain first. It's my experience that employees of medical facilities don't react well to surprises, such as you insisting on being with your loved ones while they are being prepared for a treatment. If the medical people know in advance that you're planning on being with the patient, they tend to be more accepting of your presence. Keep in mind, however, you may still have to advocate persistently to be able to do this.

You and the patient will also want to get detailed information about the test or procedure—what is going to be done? For instance, knowing what happens during a scan done by magnetic resonance imaging (MRI) can help reduce the anxiety of both you and your patient. Your patient will be required to lie perfectly still for twenty to forty minutes in a confined space with loudly banging machinery at work. You can see how that can cause a spike in stress of your patient and you as the caregiver as well. Any information that you and your patient can obtain that lessens that anxiousness will be good for both of you. Part of this procedure information-gathering needs to include information on medications that can be used to reduce anxiety, such as tranquilizers for patients undergoing MRIs. It's another way in which you can support your patients in these difficult moments.

Another set of questions to ask around a procedure or test concerns preparation. Are they to fast for some period before the procedure? When must they stop drinking liquids? Are they to take any preparatory medications? Many of the examinations of the digestive tract require enemas and other colon-clearing preparations in advance, steps that the patient is expected to take. While waiting for my sister to emerge from a treatment, I saw another patient who was expecting to have a treatment of some sort turned away because he'd just eaten a full meal. His procedure required that he not eat for six hours prior nor consume any liquids for three hours prior to the procedure. He didn't get the information, didn't understand it, or didn't take it seriously.

Conflicts between Patient and Doctor

I don't know of any patients who have begun a prolonged treatment for a disease or injury who didn't at some point find themselves in a disagreement with their doctor. It may arise out of conflicting information or treatment plans from different members of the medical team. It may arise out of a perceived lack of communication on the part of one of the medical team members. It may arise out of a perceived lack of trust of the medical team by the patients and members of their inner circle. It may be a simple case of miscommunication, in which one party thought they heard something the other party did not say. It's an inevitable part of a process that has a life-threatening condition at its core. So what do you do when it happens?

Talk it out, if possible. As we've already seen, thorough communication between the medical team and the patient—and the patient's team—is always beneficial. Here are some thoughts to keep in mind that may help defuse conflicts before they arise or to untangle them once they get started:

- *It's your loved one's body.* An obvious statement, but sometimes it needs to be reiterated. It is *his or her* body—and choice—as to what happens to it. It does not belong to anyone else, and so no one else has the privilege or responsibility of deciding what will happen to it, including the members of the medical team. This means that your loved one, and you, to some extent, needs to be absolutely clear about what will be done to his or her body and for what reason, and that you both are in concert with that course of action.

- *There are no stupid questions.* Actually there aren't even stupid answers, just confusing or incomplete ones. If you or your loved one don't understand the doctor's answer to a question, say so and ask again. Or if it's just one part of the answer you didn't understand, explain what was confusing and ask for clarification of that part.

- *Your doctor is not a saint.* This is the flipside of self-managed care. In our culture, we want to idolize the members of the life-saving professions, and doctors are first on that list, just ahead of police and firefighters. Keep in mind, however, that your loved one's doctor is a medical professional, not a professional saint. The practice of medicine involves art and intuition along with science. And it is a still-developing science. All of which means your loved one's medical team members are not miracle workers. They are human beings with some well-developed skills, which they will put to use for the benefit of your loved one. Sometimes astonishingly good results will occur. Sometimes the results will be much less than hoped for. In either extreme and all the points in between, it is a process of human endeavor, so allow for that, especially among the members of the medical team.

- *Your loved one is one of many patients.* It's important to remember this point when seeking answers to all your questions and in having the doctors respond to information that's been gathered. They may not be able to give your loved ones all the time that you or they would like. It's part of the reality of their medical practice. Many doctors will do all they can to spend as much time as possible with their patients, but the longer the visit with one patient runs, the longer the wait will be for the other patients who want to see that same doctor. Don't assume that if you get cut off it's because the doctors are rude or insensitive. They may be feeling the burden of waiting patients. It's a fine line to balance between the needs of other patients and your loved one's need to have questions answered. A word of caution: if the doctor *always* cuts the visit short and the patient and advocate feel they are not getting the answers they need, then it may be an indication you've not got a good match with the medical team, and you should be looking for a new doctor.

- *Know what the callback policy is.* One of the most frequent complaints I've heard from family and friends has been about calling their doctors' offices with a question or a request for medication and then waiting hours or even days to get a response. It's a common source of conflict between patients and the medical team. Since patients are the ones waiting for the call back, there's not a lot they can do to make it happen. A follow-up call made a few hours after the first call to remind the office staff that the patient is expecting to hear back is helpful. Repeatedly calling every hour is not going to help and will result only in alienating the doctor's support staff. These are the people you rely on, so it doesn't serve your goal of getting a response to have them angry and annoyed because of repeated calls. Before you ever have to make one of these calls to the doctor, find out what the procedure is:

  - To whom are you to talk about your questions or the patient's problems? Get to know that person on a first-name basis. It will make your phone conversations more productive and certainly friendlier.

  - Will the doctor and the other members of the medical team talk to you, the caregiver, or will they only talk to the patient?

  - Will this person or the doctor call you (or the patient) back, or are you to call him or her? If you're to call, what time is best?

  - When can you expect a call back? They will have procedures in place that cover the nature of the call, the time of day in which it's made, and the day of the week. Get to know what to expect if you call on Friday at 8:00 p.m. with a problem with the medication your loved one is taking.

- What constitutes an emergency that needs immediate attention from the medical team? This is a place for potential conflict because what feels like an emergency to you and your loved one may not be perceived as one by the medical team. Know what your options are if you feel there's a need for immediate attention and you are not getting a response.

- *Persistence is not the same as aggression.* Self-managed care is about being an informed consumer of health care services and about advocating for the patient. It's not about pounding on desks and screaming into phones to get what you think you want. Having questions answered is important to your loved ones so they can make informed choices about physicians and their treatment. Being sure to have the questions answered is key, and it's where persistence comes into play. Demanding answers or specific treatments or using any kind of threatening behavior crosses the line into aggression. If your loved ones don't feel they can get the answers or the treatment they need from a given physician, then no amount of bullying will solve that problem. At that point, it's best to find the physician who can provide the desired treatment.

Hospitals

Hospitals are a significant part of the life of anyone who has a serious medical condition. That's where tests are conducted, surgeries performed, and treatments provided. Hospitals are the home field of the medical team, and that makes patients and their supporters the away team. I have been a visitor and patient (two babies delivered and two unrelated surgeries) at my local hospital for a period of more than thirty-five years, and the place never fails to arouse negative feelings—irritation, intimidation, and fear. The hospital itself seems to grow and change overnight, so I'm constantly lost in the parking lots or the hospital corridors or in the outlying clinics, and that doesn't make my mood any less negative. Looking at the faces of the other visitors and patients, I see expressions that tell me they're not any happier about being there than I am.

This is a pretty good hospital, as hospitals go. I'm using my response to it to illustrate the point that hospitals, even the best of them, are not friendly, welcoming places where your loved ones are going to feel good just by virtue of being there. When your loved ones *are* glad to be in a hospital, you can take it as a strong indicator they are truly feeling in need of medical attention.

There are some thoughts to keep in mind when you're in whatever hospital is involved in your loved one's treatment. First, hospitals deliver treatment. That is, the institution exists as a vehicle for providing medical teams with the facilities to treat patients. This means hospitals aren't in the business of providing care. It's another one of those basic philosophical differences. The nurses, doctors, therapists, technicians, and support staff of a hospital are there to provide treatment that is designed to improve the health of their patients. They are not there, necessarily, to provide care, that is, to see to it that the patient's non-treatment needs are seen to.

For example, my sister had to have a scan of her brain through an MRI, which necessitated her being placed head-first into a very confining horizontal tube while the machine took very detailed pictures of her brain. The machine makes a terrible banging racket while it's doing its work. Imagine lying confined in a tightly enclosed space with this terrible noise all around you for forty minutes or more. She was mildly claustrophobic, and she'd gotten through the first one by sheer force of will, but it had shaken her. MaryKay told me it was as near as she'd come to having a panic attack, but she feared having the panic attack within the confined space of the tube more than she feared what was causing the panic, so she managed to force herself to stay calm.

When the medical team wanted to do another MRI just a few days later, she was terribly anxious about doing it again. The nurses and technicians were matter of fact— you have to have these pictures taken so the doctor can see what's going on in order to provide the best treatment possible. Her anxiety level didn't enter into that equation at all. That's the difference between treatment and care. Treatment requires that the scan be made, regardless of the effect on the patient. Care involves finding a way to make the treatment less stress-provoking or coming up with an alternative plan that takes into account the patient's needs.

This divergence between treatment and care also occurs in other medical institutions such as rehabilitation hospitals for patients who are too well for acute-care hospitals but not well enough for home care. The treatment/care issue can become most noticeable when the patient is dying from a long-term illness. In these instances, treatment is no longer effective, which means the staff members of the treatment facility (hospital or rehab facility) are no longer carrying out their primary function. Care at this point involves keeping the patient as comfortable as possible, something that's not usually included in the focus of treatment. Fortunately, there are more hospice and palliative care facilities available for patients in these circumstances. Palliative care, a new type of medical practice, focuses on keeping patients who are dying or suffering from chronic conditions as pain-free as possible.

Dr. M. Scott Peck, in his book *Denial of the Soul: Spiritual and Medical Perspectives on Euthanasia and Mortality,* notes the following:

> Most are now agreed that the typical modern hospital is not the best place for those who are dying from a chronic disease. A Canadian sociologist who has vividly drawn the distinction between treatment and care, points out that the primary focus of the modern hospital is treatment, and that care, perhaps of necessity, has a lower priority.[8]

Dr. Peck's opinion is supported by a study made at Georgetown University Hospital in which hidden video cameras clocked the amount of time that hospital staff and visitors spent with fifty-nine seriously ill and dying patients. The results were severe, especially taken in light of the overriding issue of the isolation that plagues patients at this stage of life. According to the study, which was published in October 2001 in the *American Journal of Medicine,* the average time of visitation over a twenty-four-hour period was seventy minutes—one hour and ten minutes for all human contact with a seriously ill or dying patient. It broke down, by average, this way:

- Attending physician—three minutes;
- Interns and residents—nine minutes;
- Nurses and nurses' aides—forty-five minutes;
- Family—thirteen minutes.

The study noted that most of the hospital staff interaction with these patients occurred in two- and three-minute intervals and that the only visits that were likely to last more than five minutes were with family. In spite of this low evidence of contact with these patients, the study showed that they actually received slightly more attention than other patients. "The good news is that [terminal] patients don't get any less time than others," said lead researcher Daniel Sulmasy, chair of ethics at St. Vincent's Manhattan Hospital and director of the Bioethics Institute of New York Medical College. "The bad news is that nobody gets [much] time."[9]

However, the good news is that more hospitals nationwide are beginning to incorporate families into their treatment plans. The most obvious way in which this is being done is to give family members unrestricted visiting hours and to issue pagers or some other notification device so that family members can be summoned if they desire to sit in on the doctors' rounds when they call on their patients who are hospitalized. The change has come about because of a dawning recognition that families are a key part of a patient's recovery process. Additionally, some hospitals have made these types of changes in realizing that the presence of a family member during a nurse's visit to provide treatment can reduce stress in the patient.[10]

The stress that staff contact can induce in patients, the limited amount of staff contact with patients, and the distinction between treatment and care should keep patients and their team on alert. *Make no assumptions* about what the hospital staff will do for your loved ones. As with the medical team, ask questions; find out who's in charge of your loved ones and who the members of that captain's team are. Many hospitals use a system in their patients' rooms in which they post the names of the people who are caring for them: the charge nurse, the floor nurse, the medication nurse, the nurse's aide, and so on. That's a good step, but you'll want to find these people, get to know them face to face, and find out where their work station is and what hours they work.

In my sister's case, every time she was hospitalized, we reacquainted ourselves with her nurses and the rest of the floor staff. But it was still MaryKay's team that got the warmed blankets or the ice chips or the other little comforting items that she needed because the nursing staff could not be relied upon to provide that level of care. When she had a significant need—pain medication, for instance—it was one of us who hunted down the nurse and brought her to the room to assess the situation. Persistence on behalf of MaryKay's needs had to be balanced with the hospital's procedures, so we did what we learned we could do to support her, doing our best not to tread on their routines. We also advocated for her when we knew what she needed was beyond what we could get for her ourselves.

Working almost outside the hospital operating system like this was a difficult choice because she and I were raised to be good little girls, to not make a fuss or disregard the rules. But there came a time when we didn't care if they thought we were good little girls or the two most aggravating women they'd ever encountered. MaryKay and her inner circle all realized that the hospital, as an institution, and its employees didn't care if she was well behaved. The level of care they were providing was all the care there was. There were many, many instances in which that fact was clearly demonstrated, including the time she suffered painful facial injuries in a fall because a hospital staff member could not be bothered to make sure she was strong enough to sit in a chair unattended. If there was to be something better for her, then we, the members of her team, were going to be the ones to provide it or insist that the hospital staff provide it. Our mission became doing whatever was necessary to ensure that she got the care she needed, along with the treatment the hospital was providing.

It is very important for patients to have an advocate for them while they are in a hospital. If they're being hospitalized for treatment, they are probably too ill to advocate for themselves. Yes, most hospitals have ombudsmen or advocates to work on behalf of patients, but the realm of these staff members primarily covers issues of treatment or compensation from health insurance or managed care systems. They are not necessarily in place to see to it that your loved one is comfortable and safe while in the hospital, so that becomes the task of the patient's team.

Of course, there's another fine line here between advocating for someone whose basic needs aren't being met and working on behalf of a patient who is angry, full of self-pity, or utterly self-centered. When your loved ones are in one of these categories, they will want to see you and the hospital staff hopping. The bed or the pillows won't be right, the room won't be warm enough or cold enough, the food will be wrong, and the nurses will be slow, stupid, or mean. You will need to decide where to draw a boundary rather than blindly wade in on the patient's behalf, no matter what the circumstance. Your job in these instances will be to find a balance between the patient's reasonable expectations and what is realistically possible for you and the hospital staff to provide.

If there is one lesson you might carry away from this chapter about supporting your loved ones in their medical treatment, it is to not make assumptions about the medical team or the treatment plan or the hospital care. Ask questions, communicate as clearly as possible, and follow up constantly.

What You Can Do

This is a reiteration of the suggestions from earlier in this chapter, listed out for easier reference:

- *Have a second person sit in on all medical appointments.* This is so important! The advocate will function as scribe and take notes, as well as prompt questions that the patient may have posed earlier to be sure they get answered by the doctor, therapist, or technician.

- *Keep a notebook and pen handy twenty-four hours a day.* You and the patient both need to keep writing materials handy to jot down questions as they occur. You *will* forget the questions if you don't write them down when they occur to you.

- *Create a team for the patient.* This would ideally come from your patients' inner circle of intimates because these will be the people who go to medical appointments with them and who assist in providing care. *Remember:* The patients are the captain of these teams, so they pick the team members and they call the plays.

- *Create a roster of the medical team members.* Include the name, specialty, phone number, address, and, if appropriate, e-mail. Include all physicians, therapists, technicians, and the pharmacists or pharmacy. The patient will need a copy of this roster and so will all the members of the patient's team.

- *Make sure everyone on both teams knows who the captain of the medical team is.* This will be the physician who is coordinating the treatments among other medical professionals and who will be the central information source. The captain is also going to be the person who resolves conflicts that may arise between members of the medical team.

- *Don't assume the medical team members know one another.* They may not know one another, so you will also be the resource for making sure they can communicate with one another. Give the roster to the members of the medical team as well as to the members of the patient's team.

- *Learn all you can about treatments, tests, and procedures prescribed for your loved ones.* These can be anxiety-producers, so it will help to know what's being called for, why it's being proposed, exactly what the process entails, and how your loved ones are expected to prepare for it. Seek permission to be at your patients' side while they are being prepared for a treatment or procedure so you can continue to function as advocate.

- *Learn the callback procedures of the medical team.* From time to time, you or your loved one will need to contact the members of the medical team by phone with questions or requests. Find out who you are to talk to on the doctor's staff and when you can expect a call back. Strive for a balance between persistence for the patient and pestering the doctor's staff.

- *Don't be shy about asking for and getting the training you need.* Patients come home from hospitals with treatment needs that the caregiver is expected to meet. This can involve changing dressings on wounds, burns, or incisions; administering injections; providing some of the necessary therapy; maintaining an intravenous system; or dealing with other medical apparatus. If you and your loved ones are going to be in that circumstance, then *before* they are released to your care, you need to be trained in dealing with the procedure. Whether the training comes from the medical team or the hospital staff, ask early, often, and clearly for the help you need to learn the procedure. Then make sure that you're allowed to practice it until you're comfortable *before* you are performing it on your own.

- *Make no assumptions.* This is a good rule for life but especially critical when you are supporting your loved one in treatment. Don't assume that one member of the medical team is communicating with another. If there's an issue that needs to be resolved, follow up to ensure resolution has taken place. This is also a vitally important rule when your loved ones are hospitalized. Make no assumptions about the care they will receive. Find out who is caring for them and what level of care is being provided. If your loved ones need more than the hospital staff provides, find a means of getting it for them. This is where the patient's team can provide significant support.

- *Suggestions for Hospital Stays*

    1. Make sure your loved ones have clothes that are practical, comfortable, and individual.

    2. Decorate their room with personal and inspirational items. Make sure the room has a view of the outside world, not a blank wall.

    3. Question authority in regard to needed tests and advocate for personal comfort for your loved one, especially during the tests.

4. Make sure the medical team is aware of the patient's unique needs and desires, be those needs dietary or more personal, such as a room with a view or the desire to listen to music just before and after surgery.

5. Make sure they have a tape, CD player, or iPod and their favorite music, meditations, or recorded books.

    My suggestion is to bring their favorites, especially music that can aid them in relaxing. Dr. Andrew Weil has produced a marvelous recording, *Sound Body, Sound Mind: Music for Healing*, which I have found to be very helpful. Beyond that, any music that does not have lyrics or is in an unknown language is also beneficial because it cannot engage the intellect and thus leaves the listener free to relax into the healing sounds.

6. Make sure your loved one will be allowed to bring the tape, iPod, or CD player into the staging area before tests or surgery, into the operating room, and into the recovery room or intensive care unit after surgery. It's a good idea to make sure permission for the player gets written into the doctor's orders.

7. Ask the surgeon and anesthesiologist to repeat positive messages to your loved ones, such as that they will awaken feeling comfortable—thirsty and hungry, for instance, as opposed to nauseous.

8. Ask the surgeon to speak to your loved one during surgery honestly, but with hope, and to repeat positive messages. Negative statements are to be absolutely avoided.

9. Arrange visits and calls from those who will nurture and provide loving support to the patient—and to you as well.

10. Help your loved ones to get moving as soon as possible after surgery. This includes walking the halls with them while they're hospitalized, as well as outside activities, such as taking them to support group meetings or for a meal out when they've been released from the hospital.[11]

LESSON SIX:
THE PATIENT

January 21, 1998

This has been an especially hard time for MaryKay. The second round of chemo, which she got six days ago, has wiped her out. She's been in bed since Monday and isn't too sure how she's going to find the strength to get to the doctor's office tomorrow. She's so devastated, physically and emotionally. And she looked so frail and sad in her bed, with her few bits of scraggly hair. We tried to make it seem like all was well, but I finally sat down on the bed and took her in my arms, and we cried. She, as she does, immediately started apologizing for her tears. I hope she gets past that soon and learns to say: "This is how I feel—take it or leave it. I'm not your good little girl. I'm a woman who might be dying, and I'm mad as hell and scared to death. Those are my feelings, and I will not hide them to try to make you feel better about this."

When we were little girls, my sister and I, with our gang of neighborhood girls, used to play hospital, in which half would take the role of nurses (never doctors, this was the fifties) and half would be patients. The patients would bravely endure their ailments while propped up on the patio furniture that we'd drag around to our long front porch. Nurses would patiently serve, usually bandaging a limb or eyes with towels or doll blankets, and a fine time was generally had passing an afternoon in our make-believe ward. Everyone wanted to be the patient, to be fussed over and then to be miraculously cured.

Right now, your life parallels the universe of our childhood game. The huge difference is that our game was make-believe. What you are experiencing now is the reality of helping care for someone who is truly suffering from a debilitating disease or a disabling injury. There are a couple of basic truths that you'll need to keep in mind over time as you support your friend, neighbor, or family member enmeshed in this unenviable circumstance:

- *In real life, no one wants to be the patient.* Your loved ones did not ask to be sick. No matter how risky their choices, they didn't choose to be injured. You will want to retain this thought because a prevailing idea in our culture blames patients for their condition. Obvious examples are smokers who are diagnosed with lung cancer. The unspoken—or even in shadow moments spoken—thought is that they are getting what they deserve. Because we all *know* cancer is a frequent outcome of smoking. Yes, they made a really bad choice when they started smoking such a dangerous and addictive substance. But it's a safe bet that when they lit that first cigarette, very few of them said to themselves, "This is great! I am going to give myself lung cancer." Becoming patients may have been the result of the behavior, but it was not the intention that motivated the behavior.

- *Your patients are not their disease or injury.* Through the denial, anger, bargaining, and depression stages of their process of acceptance, they are still the people you know and love. They remain that particular individual with whom you share a heart bond, in spite of—and because of—their faults and virtues and your shared experiences. Rabbi Kamin reminds us of this important truth in quoting from one of his friends' journals: "*Adenocarcinoma of the peritoneum,* she thought to herself. It was a cancer that had to do with her lungs. *That's what I have. But that's not who I am.*"[1]

- *You can't fix it.* This is not make-believe, and you cannot supply the miracle cures we children used to play at on our front porch. What you can do is affirm your loved ones by acknowledging that they are not guilty of causing their condition, that they are who they are and not their disease. You can provide an extremely important service to them in simply witnessing and validating what they are going through—the pain and suffering as well as the triumphs that occur along the way.

Lifestyle Impacts

Once the shock and dismay of the diagnosis has worn off, you and your patients will begin to see how the diagnosis will impact their lives. The quality of the assessment of this impact will depend on where you and your patients are in the denial stage. The greater the denial, the less the reality of their circumstance is going to be recognized. And that's okay for a time. Denial is a very useful tool that allows us to ease into dealing with shocking new events—a kind of protective blanket we can keep wrapped around us until we've adjusted to the cold reality of the circumstances. But at some point, you and your loved ones are going to have to start dealing with these changes that have the potential to affect the most fundamental aspects of life—everything from finances to career to living arrangements to sex drive.

The financial impact can come from a variety of sources, the cost of medical treatment and the quality of the health insurance coverage, if any, being the most obvious. Even the best quality health insurance still generates expenses for people who are undergoing medical treatment. It also creates a huge mountain of paperwork that the patients or caregivers are going to have to manage. It's been my personal experience that there are always issues with health insurance—treatments, doctors' visits, or hospital stays which are denied payment, leading to debate between doctor and patient on one side and the insurance company on the other. Dealing with insurance is a difficult and stress-inducing job. There are also related impacts, such as the expense of special equipment or trained caregivers.

Loss of income from the inability to work is one effect, but that comes tied to a deeper identity loss if your loved ones can no longer work or are forced by their condition to take a different job. Our jobs are a huge piece of our identity, and that can be a significant loss. A change in living arrangements is another one of those two-edged impacts. Having to move out of your home has personal identity impacts as well as financial consequences.

Loss of physical intimacy between patients and their spouses or partners gets added into the mix in a variety of ways. It may be the direct result of the injury or medical condition, it could be among the side effects of the treatment, or it could come from the stress of the total experience. The good news is that this problem can be temporary, particularly if it comes from side effects or stress. Once those circumstances resolve themselves, there's a good chance that the libido can return to its normal levels.

In dealing with these kinds of impacts, the first step is to recognize which ones will affect your loved one. It may be minor, the "speed bump in the road of life" that my sister experienced in her initial cancer treatments. The surgery and subsequent chemotherapy inhibited her ability to work, but for just a few months. She had an excellent medical plan, so the economic impact of her first bout was limited. Obviously there was an impact on her sex life after a mastectomy and during the course of the nausea-inducing chemo, but it was all relatively short-lived, lasting less than six months.

If your patients' conditions are chronic—for instance, if they're heart, dementia, or dialysis patients, if they've suffered a spinal cord or traumatic brain injury, or if they are dealing with a central nervous system disease—then these impacts are going to be long-lasting, if not permanent. In those kinds of circumstances, a new way of life needs to be found, and that can pose either an opportunity or a threat, depending on how you and your loved ones choose to view the situation.

There's a business management assessment technique called SWOT—strengths, weaknesses, opportunities, and threats. It's a way of deciding on a course of action by listing factors that apply under each heading. If you're stuck, unable to act in the stress of the moment, you might give it a try. The idea is to make a comprehensive list of what you've got to work with—the SWOTs—and then come up with a plan that maximizes the strengths and opportunities and minimizes the weaknesses and threats.

There is no magic wand for dealing with life impacts of the illness or injury. There is simply the necessity of recognizing the degree to which the condition of your loved ones is going to affect their lifestyle and then making whatever adjustments are possible. This is not a simple process because of the medical condition with which you are dealing. Your loved ones are facing a life-threatening illness or are in pain from an injury. There are medical issues in the treatment of their condition. They are working through the emotional stages to acceptance, and on top of all of that, they have these lifestyle impacts to face. This is where active listening and affirmations are *so* important. Outside assistance with these fundamental impacts is also very important and can prove most helpful.

You may be able to see the path they should take—or at least you think it's the path they should take—but it's *their* medical problem and it's *their* life, and I urge you to be extremely cautious about forcing your ideas onto their process. For example, I did not like the oncologist that both my father and sister had chosen. Regardless of my feelings about his problematic personality, they trusted him completely. The best I could do was to urge a second opinion be obtained. My dad didn't get one. My sister did and was more convinced than ever that her oncologist was the right choice. I'd voiced my opinion one time to each of them. After that, my job was to support them in their choice.

Spouses or life partners are in a precarious situation because they are deeply affected too, in many of the same ways that the patients are. You can see why Dr. Kubler-Ross stressed the importance of communication, the necessity of being able to express feelings and share thoughts and ideas. There's a very fine line between effective problem solving through mutual communication and taking control of someone else's life, be they the patient or the patient's spouse or partner.

Side Effects

Side effects are those outcomes which result from treatment that have nothing to do with the results the treatment is intended to provide. Broken eggs could be said to be a side effect of making an omelet. It's such an innocuous-sounding term, and yet it can carry such a terrible reality. How many times in those televised ads for prescription medicines have you *really* heard what they say about side effects—may cause sudden bleeding, may cause nausea and vomiting, may cause a whole host of things that we all tend to ignore because we're so focused on the cure that's being offered.

There are two truths about side effects. First, all treatments—surgery, drugs, dialysis, lung treatments, any and all of it—produce side effects. Second, when someone is receiving treatment for a serious condition, rest assured that the side effects are going to be equally serious. They can't be ignored, and in fact, they will become the center of attention because of the suffering they cause. It's so easy to mentally minimize what side effects are going to do to your loved one. After all, this person is being treated for a serious, even life-threatening illness. Why worry about a little thing like side effects? The medical team often will touch lightly on side effects for the same reason—they're focused on curing the disease through treatments. To them, side effects are just that, something that occurs on the side, out of their frame of reference. It's easy for them to regard these very physical circumstances this way since they're not the ones experiencing them or living with them every day.

The following is a very mild example:

My friend Elizabeth was diagnosed with breast cancer. She had a lumpectomy to remove the small tumor and then began a course of radiation treatments. Whether she was not told or whether she failed to hear the information, she was not prepared for any side effects other than perhaps a bit of fatigue after a few weeks of treatments. "You're powering down the water, right?" I asked when she was telling me about starting the radiation. She looked puzzled. Bless her, she took my suggestion to drink lots of water, but the next time we met, about two weeks later, she mentioned that constipation was a problem. I suggested she ask her doctor for a stool softener. The point I want to make is not my knowledge but the fact that Elizabeth was unprepared for these very common side effects of radiation treatments.

I suspect we all have a tendency to view side effects as being temporary. Blessedly, most are, but some are not.

When my sister was receiving radiation treatments for brain tumors after her cancer recurred, one of the side effects was that more than the tumors were burned by the radiation. The sheath of tissue that wrapped the nerve bundles that carried auditory messages between her left ear and the temporal lobe of her brain was damaged as well. The result was that she initially experienced a loud static-like noise in her head, an extremely disruptive and unpleasant sensation that was constantly with her. It eventually died off after the treatments ceased, but the end result was a substantial loss of hearing in that ear. This condition never improved, and she spent the last six months of her life with a hearing aid.

The hearing loss was never discussed with her and her husband, nor was it brought up when I went with her to medical appointments. As distressing as this loss was to her, I think she was most upset by not being prepared for it. The lesson for both caregivers and patients is to not only ask in detail about side effects (see the list below) but ask also if any of them have the potential to become permanent.

You and your loved ones should be prepared by the medical team for side effects, whatever the treatment they're undergoing. This is why two-person medical visits are so important. Ask your doctors about *all* potential side effects and get detailed answers about what they are likely to be and how the distress they cause can be minimized or at least reduced.

What follows is a preliminary list for you to take to the medical team. It includes a bit of information about each side effect. Go down the checklist with the doctor to be sure you've got an idea of what to expect and how to deal with it. Ask if the treatment proposed for your loved ones will produce side effects that *aren't* on this list. What else can they anticipate as side effects? What are some preventatives that your patients can engage in? What activities or foods should they absolutely avoid? Don't hesitate to get more information from your medical team until you're satisfied that you know what to expect and how to cope with it.

In some cases, the medications used to treat side effects will themselves produce side effects. This is true of pain medications, as well as drugs used to treat the side effects of chemotherapy. In those instances, the side effects (from the meds to treat side effects) can include dizziness, drowsiness, dry mouth, blurred vision, constipation, and nausea. Ask the doctor any time a treatment or medication is proposed or prescribed: "What are the side effects going to be, and how can we work to minimize them?" That question applies to treatments given to lessen the impact of side effects, as well as the side effects themselves.

- Hair loss—This is most common in chemotherapy because the poisons used in chemo are ones that attack the quickly reproducing tumor cells. They attack *all* of the body's quickly reproducing cells, including the hair follicles. I don't know of any cancer patients who haven't seized upon the fact that in a few rare cases people get through chemo without losing some or all of their hair. Personally, I don't know a case where the hair loss hasn't occurred. Keep in mind that we are hairy creatures, and your loved ones will lose *all* of their hair—body hair, eyebrows, eyelashes, nose hair, pubic hair, and facial hair. They will look a bit like a baby, except that even babies have a sort of downy body hair. The good news is that it will all grow back in after the treatments are over and the poison has left their body. Sometimes the first crop can be of a strange texture and color compared to what the patient had before the treatments started. That first growth eventually falls out naturally and is replaced by the patient's normal hair.

- Loss of fingernails and toenails—This is caused because the chemo poisons get stuck in some parts of the body, such as the fine vascular system in fingers and toes. The buildup kills off the cells that grow fingernails and toenails. This makes some ordinary tasks, such as opening bottles with caps, especially prescriptions in bottles with childproof caps, very difficult.

- Nausea—This is a common side effect of many medical treatments, including chemo as well as use of pain medications following surgeries and for chronic conditions. In its most mild form, it may involve a simple loss of appetite. When it's severe, the patient may not be able to keep any food down. Doctors can prescribe medications to offset the nausea, but sometimes it's tricky getting people who feel like they're going to throw up—or who may be having a spell of vomiting—to take and keep down additional medication. That's when you can ask for suppositories or injectable meds, but keep in mind it will be you who is administering these drugs. Nausea at this level obviously also affects your loved one's desire, and therefore ability, to eat. When they say no to a proffered food, take them at their word, and do your best to find something that appeals to them, no matter how strange it may seem to you.

- Constipation, diarrhea, and other gastric problems—Digestive problems are a side effect of many kinds of treatments and medications. They can cause embarrassment to your loved ones if they can't control their digestive problems, so you want to be sensitive to their desire to not be in public or even around many people—perhaps even you. They may be experiencing significant pain from this side effect, so it's not helpful to dismiss these problems as being on par with a gas attack or tummy rumbles.

- Mouth sores or sores elsewhere on the body—One side effect of chemo is mouth sores, which also obviously contribute to a patient's inability to eat. Bedsores (also known as pressure sores), for patients who are confined to bed, are another significant problem. In both cases—particularly with bedsores—the sores present an opportunity for infection, so they need to be taken seriously and treated early and carefully. The actor/director Christopher Reeves, paralyzed following a riding accident, died of a severe infection that began in a pressure sore. Be watchful for sores whether your loved one is permanently bedridden or merely confined while recovering from surgery.

- Burns, internal and/or external—Radiation therapy has come a long way since my mother was treated with it in 1964, when she was left with a deep, red burn mark on the skin on her chest, neck, and shoulder. However, as in the case of my sister's hearing loss, current-day radiation treatments still hold the potential for great unintended impact. Ask your doctor about other organs that might be affected by any radiation treatments. Reproductive organs can be damaged, as can bone marrow. I believe that my dad's blood condition was the result of the radiation treatments he'd been given for both his primary cancer as well as the secondary lymphoma. Be aware that permanent external skin burns, like my mother's, can still occur, even after forty years of technological improvements. Physicians will sometimes dismiss this side effect as being nothing more than just a bad case of sunburn. You need to know how bad it might be. This "bad case of sunburn" can affect your patients' appearance, and that can have a damaging effect on their psychological and emotional state.

- Lymphedema—This is a condition that results from surgical removal of lymph nodes, injury to them in an accident, or damage to them from radiation treatments. The loss or malfunctioning of the nodes allows for an accumulation of the lymph fluid that the lymphatic channels disperse throughout the body. This accumulation produces swelling in the nearest extremity. It's uncomfortable for patients and can lead to more serious medical conditions. Because it affects their appearance, it can have an emotional as well as physical impact.

- Weight loss or weight gain—When patients are suffering from digestive problems as a result of their treatment, they will likely lose weight. In our diet-conscious culture, this may seem like a blessing; but our bodies need nutrition to be able to overcome disease or injury, so this is not necessarily a good thing. Likewise, some drugs such as steroids used to treat chronic pain and inflammation can cause weight gain, an emotionally painful consequence for some people. More than the weight itself, to patients, this side effect represents a fundamental loss of control over their own body—their ability to control their weight, either loss or gain. The effect on their self-image can be significant. Mary Susan Herczog, the *Los Angeles Times* reporter who put on weight as a result of cancer treatment, which also caused her to lose her hair, was concerned that her struggle would go unnoticed in the shock of seeing her "bald and fat...they are going to think, *Boy, Mary's really let herself go to hell.*" [2]

- Infertility/loss of libido—The infertility can be voluntary, as in the case of breast cancer patients who do not want to risk the free flow of estrogen that a pregnancy would create. By voluntary, I mean that patients voluntarily elect to become infertile rather than risk a recurrence of their disease. Or it can be involuntary, such as the loss of libido or function in some heart, stroke, or prostate and testicular cancer patients. It can result from surgery, chemotherapy, or radiation treatments. It is an issue for people with spinal injuries and central nervous system disorders. It can have a significant impact, in part because of what it may mean in terms of loss of identity—they are no longer the man or woman they once were by virtue of their infertility. But it also can mean a far greater loss if it involves a loss of sexual function, a loss of intimacy. Your loved ones may feel isolated because of their medical condition, and the loss of the closeness of a physical relationship may only deepen that feeling.

- Hot flashes/chills—Our bodies are amazing machines. When we have to start tinkering with various mechanisms in order to treat a disease or injury, whether it's with drugs, chemotherapy, radiation, or surgery, some of the mechanisms are going to get out of whack. The body's ability to regulate temperature is important to your loved ones' physical comfort. Going through their day in a hot, sweating state or wrapped in layers of sweaters is not fun. The underlying issue, aside from the very real physical discomfort, is about loss of control over one's body, as it is with weight-related issues and loss of fertility or sexual function. It packs a big emotional impact.

- Dryness—Like many of these side effects, dryness can come from any source of treatment. It can be severe enough to cause painful cracking and bleeding of the skin, a danger because of the opportunity for infection. Dryness in the eyes can cause chronic eye irritation and make it impossible for patients to wear their contact lenses. Do they have a pair of glasses that will provide the vision correction they need if this happens? Loss of saliva can lead to dental problems. Severe dryness can also impact sexuality. Fortunately, there are shelves in pharmacies full of lubricants and moisturizers available to help offset this side effect.

- Seizures—Anyone with a neurological condition, either as a result of disease or injury, is at risk for seizures. An acquaintance, whose sister had started experiencing seizures as a result of brain surgery, became impatient with the doctors who told her sister that she should be glad to be alive and not to be distressed about the seizures. The woman couldn't drive and or even go for a walk by herself. Travel became problematic, as did her former athletic interests. The impact for her was significant. Keep in mind that seizures can also have a huge impact in your loved one's life. As a caregiver, be sure you know what to do in the event your loved one has a seizure. Ask your loved one's doctor for the information you need.

- Tenderness or loss of feeling in hands and/or feet (neuropathy)—This is another result of chemotherapy poisons attacking quickly growing cells. The following anecdote is from *Speak the Language of Healing:* "His mouth, hands, and feet had a serious delayed reaction [after chemotherapy]. They became so sore and tender, he was not able to hold his own fork or walk across the floor... he could neither swallow nor chew."[3] Numbness can also be a result, and it can last for several months after chemo is over. It can also be permanent. Diabetes patients suffer from a variation of this problem when their circulatory systems don't work well. Dialysis is another treatment that produces numbness, but most often of the mouth, making it difficult to eat.

Think of how difficult it is to manage your mouth after having a cavity filled at the dentist, and you can understand what a dialysis patient is dealing with.

- Effect on the other senses: vision, hearing, smell, and taste—This can include having a bad reaction to a drug, especially a painkiller, which could cause visual or auditory hallucinations. All forms of treatment, surgery, chemo, and drugs have an ability to affect our body's sensors. Jan Stillman, the family friend who underwent chemo for lung cancer, struggled for months with the fact that around the time of her chemo infusion everything smelled and tasted like tin.

- Effect on blood—Many drugs have effects on blood production. For example, chemo may affect the production of red or white cells in the blood. Sometimes drugs can be used to treat this problem. Sometimes blood transfusions are necessary to correct the problem. Radiation and the severe chemo treatments that are used in instances of bone marrow harvesting or bone marrow transplants can depress or stop the body's ability to make and sustain normal blood counts. Additionally, drugs used for treating a wide variety of diseases—such as anti-seizure medications—can reach toxic levels in a patient's blood, necessitating constant monitoring and adjusting of these medications.

- Effect on memory and concentration—My sister-in-law, Rosemarie, said that the other chemo patients whom she saw regularly at the City of Hope in Southern California had a series of standing jokes about their loss of concentration and memory because of the treatments they were receiving. This condition is widely known as "chemo brain." They all knew what recent studies verify—some treatments affect memory and concentration. One study conducted at Dartmouth University focused on the ability of patients receiving chemo for breast cancer or lymphoma to perform simple concentration tasks. The results, not surprisingly, were that chemo patients couldn't concentrate at their normal levels. Another study released in early 2001 showed short-term memory loss in heart or lung patients who had undergone surgeries in which they were hooked up to artificial heart/lung machinery. The implications are significant for either group of patients. Those who want to carry on through chemo as if it were no big deal, or who are forced to stay at their jobs during these treatments, and those who want to get back to normal as quickly as possible after transplant or other surgery may become depressed over their loss of these fundamental abilities. They need to know that it's not them, it's the side effect.

• Fatigue—This may sound like the least problematic of this list, but for those who suffer from it, this is an extremely debilitating side effect. Patients awaken from a long night's sleep feeling as if they haven't slept at all. They lose the ability to get to their jobs; keep up with routine chores, such as paying bills or preparing meals; or even engage in enjoyable leisure activities. Just getting to and from a medical appointment may become an enormous trial for someone suffering from this level of fatigue. It can be part of a severe depression, or it can trigger an episode of depression.

- Severe itching—This can be a result of severely dry skin, or it can be a nervous system reaction to a variety of drugs. Dialysis patients can suffer from this side effect. Patients who suffer from this side effect can scratch themselves to the point of bleeding, and that, in turn, is an opportunity for infection.

- Involuntary movement of the extremities—This is not a seizure but the sometimes severe twitching of hands, feet, or head that is commonly experienced by dialysis patients. Any loss of control over a patient's body causes distress.

- Side effects from the medications taken to treat side effects. For instance, thrush (candida albicans) is an infection of the mouth, throat, or tongue that can result from taking certain anti-nausea medications. Those medications are regularly prescribed to offset the effects of pain medications or chemotherapy.

Emotional and Spiritual Impacts

"Why me?"

This question inevitably comes up as patients move through their medical treatment. You are probably going to ask the same question from time to time. It's natural to ask, but keep in mind that *there is no answer.* The medical team may be able to supply some sort of hint that relates to genetic predisposition to a specific disease or a lifestyle that may lead to a greater risk for certain disease, but none of those factors can ever answer the question of why your loved ones have been afflicted with their particular condition at this particular time. Accepting that reality is part of what you and your loved one are processing through the five stages of Dr. Kubler-Ross.

Knowing this is a normal part of the emotional processing that surrounds an illness or injury may not, in itself, lessen the necessity for answering the question. The arrival of the disease or injury is an utterly capricious event, yet in our rational culture, we want to find a cause for it. Since there is no answer in terms of our day-to-day lives, we look to forces beyond us for an explanation:

- It's karma.

- I'm working out an issue from a past life.

- God is testing me.

These possibilities are as unanswerable as the role of genetics or lifestyle, so once again, patients are left with uncertainty, even mystery, as to why they are in the condition they are in. And that's all there truly is. The disease or injury simply is. *Why* it is doesn't matter as much as acceptance of the *fact of it.* Carol Matzkin Orsborn, one of the co-authors of *Speak the Language of Healing,* notes:

> At these times you must have the courage to confront the possibility that what happened to you or to others contains no inherently useful meaning whatsoever. Sometimes the only lesson to be gleaned is that life brings with it no guarantees. Things don't always make sense. They are not always deserved. In the end, all we can know for certain is the mystery. We must look elsewhere than the illusion of personal power to find meaning in the midst of suffering.[3]

So you and your loved one are going to be left with *the* question ultimately unanswered, which is not comforting while you both are struggling to come to acceptance. And while that process is going on, there are other issues that need to be faced, such as the impacts on lifestyle. If your loved ones were independent people before their illness or injury, then the degree to which they've lost that independence will deeply affect their emotional state. For some, this may not become an issue.

For instance, take cancer patients who are undergoing an initial course of treatment that promises to have them in a state of remission in a short period, perhaps just a few months. The loss of independence may not be experienced for more than a few days of downtime during chemotherapy or just after surgery. However, when the condition is debilitating and long-term, then loss of independence becomes a much more significant factor.

My sister, MaryKay, was a very independent woman. After the recurrence of her cancer, with the severe radiation and chemotherapy treatments for her brain tumors, she became completely, and very reluctantly, dependent on others. She could not drive and finally needed to use a walker to move around. Common activities such as grocery shopping or even getting the dog food off the top of the refrigerator had to be turned over to someone else. She hated it. Whenever we went anywhere together, she'd try to weasel out of taking the walker along. But knowing that she risked injury from a fall due to her unsteadiness, it was by far the kindest thing I could do to insist that she bring it and use it. She didn't always see that insistence as being an act of kindness, so I framed it in terms of my personal comfort level. It wasn't "bring the walker because you *have to* use it." I said and sincerely meant "bring the walker because *I'll feel better* knowing that you're using it."

So many of the people I know who've had a serious illness hate being turned into a needy person by their condition. They are generally the people who have always supported family and friends whenever there was a need, and to find themselves as the recipient of support is uncomfortable for them.

Dad was a classic example. He *was not* going to let anyone—other than his wife—know how sick he was in the last months of his life. He had always been the tower of strength for everyone else, and he intended to continue in that role. He managed to get into the office and to meetings to continue his life's work. He simply refused to give up and to let people know the severity of his condition. In doing so, he got to live out his time on his terms, which meant accepting very little help from anyone. It was a big step when he quit driving and allowed others to chauffeur him to medical appointments or business meetings.

I suspect that this need *not* to be needy comes from a couple of sources. In our free enterprise world, to need help from anyone is to be considered weak, a pitiable state. It also has to do with control of one's life, the quintessence of independence. Physician Dale A. Matthews, in his book *The Faith Factor: Proof of the Healing Power of Prayer*, says,

> [A serious medical condition] presents a spiritual crisis, a crisis of meaning. As long as we are well, we can remain relatively independent, and we can gain feelings of self-worth and purpose from our work in the world ... Once serious illness strikes ... we can no longer derive our self-esteem from our accomplishments; we may no longer even be able to care for our own bodies.[4]

Our culture values people who are both in control of their own lives, the captains of their fates, and who do not need help from anyone else. Yet American culture has always presented a dichotomy on the issue of neediness. From the days of the Pilgrims to the Great Depression, we have put a high value on helping one another. A barn raising wasn't seen as an act of charity—it was an act of community.

Like the glass that's either half-full or half-empty, it's a matter of perspective. Your loved ones may see themselves in a negative light as being needy. Or they may see themselves as being the recipient of the caring that they've given others, now coming back to them. The perspective can shift as they move toward the acceptance stage, being able to accept that their condition simply *is* without having to find a cause for it and then being able to accept the loving care that you and other intimates have to offer.

Self-sabotage

Understanding how these impacts and side effects affect your loved ones is a good start. Beyond the point of understanding, it is the patients who are responsible for integrating the information into their lives. It will be your loved ones, not you, who must follow doctor's orders or advice on ways to mitigate the effects of treatment, and it must be the patients who make the decisions about how to cope with lifestyle impacts. Turning information into an action plan doesn't always happen smoothly. Your loved ones have a denial phase to work through, and if it's still in place when treatments start, bringing on side effects, they may not engage in behaviors that are beneficial, or they may resist incorporating changes in their lifestyle necessitated by their condition.

When my father was given radiation treatment following removal of a cancerous testicle in 1991, he absolutely ignored his doctor's advice on what to avoid eating and drinking and what to be sure to include in his diet. At the end of the six-week course of treatments, he was hospitalized with severe dehydration, brought on by painful gastric problems. His intestines were severely irritated by the radiation. Dad was an absolutely horrid patient during that hospitalization, angry and rude to everyone in the hospital. I believe that part of his emotional reaction to his physical state was out of anger at himself, that he'd had a hand in bringing about his distressful condition.

Would it have been any different if he'd followed doctor's orders? I don't know, but I do know that when he was being treated for the secondary cancer that occurred six years later, he was scrupulous about drinking the large amounts of recommended water and avoiding all the foods and activities put on the banned list by his doctor. The result was that there were no hospitalizations or accompanying angry, rude behavior.

Why do our loved ones engage in this kind of self-sabotage? It's about denial. Facing the reality of a life-threatening condition or permanent disability is hard because it forces each of us to confront our own mortality. In these circumstances of illness or injury, we are looking at the inevitability of death, whether it's as a direct result of the medical condition or if it is something more remote in time. The response of the human psyche is denial as a form of protection against this shocking reality. This rejection of our own mortality is a very real force in all lives, regardless of age or culture. It is a fundamental part of the human condition. Recall Dr. Peck's summary of Freud's understanding of the life force, or Eros, that I mentioned earlier.

As caregivers, we too are confronting issues of our own mortality and have our own phase of denial to work through. Sometimes, if we're still in denial, we will enable our loved one's self-sabotage. Or it may be that our patients are clear about adopting new behaviors to take into account their change of lifestyle and treatment, but we, the caregivers, are working to undermine that. We offer a glass of wine when it's on the forbidden list. We argue against moving to a wheelchair accessible home. We can't find something supportive to say about the new wig or wardrobe that accommodates the prosthesis or colostomy bag. As caregivers, our role is to support, and if we can't do that because of our own issues, then we need to take a step back and find a way to work through our issues so that it will permit us to provide the help that our loved ones need.

Time With the Patient

There are some common sense approaches you can take in spending time with your loved ones. As I have mentioned previously, your greatest gift to them is your willingness and ability to engage in active listening, to let them express their feelings. Rabbi Kamin recommends that we let our patients set the tone of our encounters with them. "The person you are visiting will usually set the tone; his or her condition has already set the agenda."[5]

A sense of humor can be a great tool for both of you. If the patient is someone who enjoyed laughter before his illness or injury, humor can be a means of optimism and intimacy. Again, let the patient lead. Someone who is distressed over a change in his physical appearance isn't gong to want you cracking jokes about it.

My mother's longtime friendship with Jan Stillman nearly ended when Mom was undergoing chemo treatments that left her bald. One day, when Jan dropped by the house, she decided to create some laughs by pulling Mom's wig off her head. Mom was not laughing; even though just the two of them were present, Mom was humiliated. Jan remembered that incident with sad irony several years later when hair loss from her chemotherapy forced her to wear a wig.

It's a boundary issue, and patients need to set the boundaries. However, if they're willing to include humor in their process, allowing for shared laughter, then you will have a special bond with them.

My mother had a prosthetic breast that she used—actually a series of them—following her radical mastectomy in 1964. She was sensitive to the lymphedema that resulted from the surgery, as well as the somewhat-altered appearance of her whole shoulder and chest area, even with the prosthesis in place. But she always took the process of trying on clothes, especially bathing suits, with a good dose of humor. When I was along on these outings, her good humor made me feel included in her innermost circle, a part of her team. That feeling of being part of the team was extremely important to me because of the occasional information blackouts that she and Dad would impose.

My sister wanted to be prepared for the hair loss from her second round of chemotherapy, so we went wig shopping. The first time around, she'd decided to use scarves, and so she never bothered with a wig. But the chemo treatments after her recurrence were going to be lengthy and severe, and she decided a wig would be a good idea.

Once we got into the wig shop, she began to play with the variety of colors and styles. She had jaw-length, dark-red, thick and curly hair, and we had a great time playing with new looks for her—long, blonde hair or short, black hair. You name it, she tried it on. We laughed heartily about some of the results and got some new ideas from others. It was great fun! She later confessed that the reason she hadn't used a wig in her first chemo was that she had so dreaded having to shop for one. "But you made it fun," she told me. Laughter definitely took the sting out of the experience for her.

One last thought on the subject of your time with the patient. It's not always going to be fun and laughter-filled. There are going to be trying times too. To the three caveats with which I opened this lesson, I add a fourth:

- *Your loved ones are not in this condition just to make your life difficult.* That seems an obvious statement, but there will be times when you're going to find that thought creeping into your consciousness. Don't buy into it. They didn't do it just to complicate their life or yours. And don't feel guilty because you've had that thought. It's absolutely normal because your life *has* changed. The process of adjusting to that change, whether it's permanent or temporary, isn't easy. My best advice when you find yourself in this spot is to figure out what's bothering you—what the demand or circumstance is that irritates you—and see what can be done to either make it less irritating or to make it possible for you to accept it without it carrying the sting that it has.

Healthy and Helpful Behaviors

One important way to care for your loved ones will be to support them in their lifestyle changes and healthy behaviors that are recommended as part of their treatment. The process they are engaged in is hard enough; the idea is for you both to find ways in which to create some ease within it.

Think of what you can do for them as being part of their team. They have a huge assignment facing them in dealing with their medical condition, and it may feel overwhelming to them. As a member of their support team, your job will be to help reduce the overwhelming quality to what lies ahead for them. You can do this by taking a one-piece-at-a-time approach so they don't feel like they have to do it all, do it all at once, or do it by themselves. It can offer great comfort to them to know that while they've got the big piece of overcoming or coping with their disease or injury, they can rely on you to back them up on the myriad of details which surround their central effort.

Sometimes it's the little things that can be most meaningful to a patient. One of my sister's close friends, Pam Trowe, provided incredible support for MaryKay when she had resumed chemotherapy following the recurrence of her cancer. MaryKay knew she was going to lose the hair that had grown back just six months before, following her first series of treatments. She didn't want to watch it fall out and told Pam how much she was going to hate the process of losing it again. So Pam called a friend who runs a barbershop in a nearby town and set up an after-hours appointment. She went with MaryKay to the shop, where the owner waited with the shades drawn. With Pam holding her hand, MaryKay had her head shaved. Pam's wonderful gift was in helping MaryKay take control of this inevitable side effect of her treatments and doing it with the privacy that provided my sister with the greatest level of comfort possible.

There are innumerable little things you can do for your loved ones. For instance, many patients cannot get in and out of bathtubs because of their physical condition. But showers can be problematic too, especially if they are very weak. Putting a stool in a shower is usually recommended. But if you think about it, stools are a long way down and can be difficult for your loved one to sit down on and then get up from. What about using one of those cheap plastic outdoor chairs or low tables? They are higher than a stool and easier for someone who is physically impaired to use. (Just be sure to put some no-skid material onto the feet so it won't slide in the wet shower.) Take the idea a step further and look at what the needs are as they are drying off and getting dressed. They may need a chair or bench in the bathroom, as well as the chair in the shower.

One of the things you can do for your loved ones is to encourage them to provide themselves with care. Carol Matzkin Orsborn, one of four authors of *Speak the Language of Healing,* talks about the need for patients to treat themselves gently:

> Common sense...would suggest that when your body is ill, you need rest. I'm not talking about becoming a couch potato, giving up and going into hiding. But I am suggesting that we all need balance in our lives: times when we are driving ourselves through the force of will, and times when we are nurturing ourselves by letting go and relaxing deeply. This is true for all of us, and doubly true for people dealing with serious illness.[8]

Here are some practical suggestions:

Encourage your patients to take their physicians' recommendations seriously. The list of side effects is harrowing, but there are ways in which some of those side effects can be at least mitigated by behavior changes. If the doctor recommends drinking two liters of water a day, then you can support your loved ones by helping them with a plan to achieve that goal.

In early 1998, when my sister was starting her chemo treatments for the recurrence of her cancer, she became bedridden by the debilitating nausea the treatments created. She ultimately had to be briefly hospitalized because of severe dehydration. She got into bed feeling so nauseous and so weak that she couldn't manage to walk down the long hallway to her kitchen to get the needed water or juice. Tap water in our area has a bad taste, and so she didn't want to drink from her close-by bathroom sink.

Dad and I decided that the solution would be to buy her a flat-topped cooler and have her husband set it up by her bed before he left for work in the morning. It kept her much-needed water and juices close at hand, which enabled her to stay hydrated and yet rest as comfortably as possible. We included a thermos so she could keep her herbal tea hot. Obviously, what we were dealing with in the first instance of the dehydration was, in part, her very understandable denial. She said later that our action on her behalf helped her to realize that she needed to be more proactive in taking care of herself.

Mary Susan Herczog, in her series of articles in the *Los Angeles Times*, detailed her experiences of surgery and chemotherapy treatments for breast cancer. Her recollection of her weekly visits to a Chinese herbalist to lessen the side effects of the chemo include some humor:

> She also prescribed a strict diet, banning, among other things, fried, smoked, or spicy foods, garlic, dairy products, sugar, white flour, and yes, chocolate. But hey, I can have all the seaweed, brown rice, and mushrooms I want.
>
> Right, I said. I'm going to go nine months without chocolate. You know what? I'm not going to go nine hours without it.[9]

The patient *does* need an occasional taste of a favorite dish or comfort food, even if it's not recommended. Keep in mind that an occasional piece of chocolate is not going to be harmful in the same way that a steady diet would—even if you're not undergoing treatment.

Meals need to support the treatment plan. All serious illnesses bring with them a restricted diet—there are some foods that just aren't healthy for people with heart disease, with specific conditions that affect internal organs, or who are undergoing chemotherapy. Take the doctor's recommendations seriously and support your loved ones by not presenting them with banned foods—don't buy them if you're doing the grocery shopping, and don't prepare them in a meal. As Ms. Herczog noted, that may mean your loved one has to give up on chocolate. While hers was a humorous take on the subject, there are some patients, such as diabetes patients and those on dialysis, for whom even a small deviation from a prescribed diet can produce disastrous results, so don't tempt them.

In addition to taking seriously the dietary restrictions, patients may need to change their eating habits. For some, this may mean giving up on three large meals a day in favor of several smaller ones. Dietitians tell us that four to six small snacks over the course of the day is actually better for our digestive system than three large meals. Look at the break from the habitual meal plan as an opportunity to find new ways to prepare, present, and eat meals together. Shifting your attitude will help your loved ones make the changes their health requires.

You'll notice that some suggestions for supporting patients involve giving them comfort foods or other special treats, like Ms. Herczog's occasional piece of chocolate. This is one of many balancing acts that you are going to have to learn. On the one hand, you have the weight of the medical condition and the dietary restrictions that it imposes on your loved one. On the other hand, you have the necessity to provide loving care by providing a certain level of pampering. Which one carries more weight? Together, you and the patient will have to decide how to answer that question. For some of you, the restriction is absolute and cannot be violated even once with out serious repercussions. For others, the occasional treat of a banned food, like chocolate, won't pose a serious problem.

Encourage the patient to let go of social obligations. During treatment, even if it's just a light dose of radiation or recovery from outpatient surgery, up through the more severe treatments, social activity is a detriment. The human body needs to be quiet in order to heal, so now is not the time for your loved ones to convince the world that they are perfectly all right by maintaining active work or social schedules. Work can't always be avoided, but it's a good idea to cut back as much as possible. And the social engagements need to be suspended to allow for recuperation. There will always be parties and meetings to attend. Giving it a rest for a few weeks or months is a great assist in the recovery process. As that noted twentieth century philosopher, Leroy Robert "Satchel" Paige, observed: "The social ramble ain't restful."

My friend Archie had a full life as a well-respected venture capitalist, a well-liked golfing member of the local country club, and a nationally sought-after board member in both the for-profit and not-for-profit world. He loved the symphony, and he regularly traveled to the east coast to visit his children and grandchildren while attending to business. When his prostate cancer returned and he was put into a course of chemotherapy treatments, he dropped all of his outside activities—he retired from his business, he resigned from the many boards of directors on which he served, and he gave up all evening engagements.

"I am cutting out anything that might resemble stress," he told me. "I've got enough stress with the cancer. I don't need anything else added to that."

Exercise is one way patients can ease the stress of their treatment. I'm not talking aerobics here. There are ways to exercise that stretch the muscles and give patients a way of relieving stress. Walking is excellent. This shouldn't be a power walk in which the goal is to cover as much ground as quickly as possible. A more beneficial walk would be an easy stroll through a scenic area of a park, which will afford patients an opportunity to let go of the stress of the medical circumstance and enjoy the beauty of the surroundings. "Easy does it" should be the guiding principle. Some of the meditative Asian exercises, such as yoga and t'ai chi chuan, can be a wonderful means of getting exercise while relaxing through a meditative state. Archie became a regular at the local yoga classes and followed those sessions with a couple of quiet hours with a book on his patio.

Some treatments will leave your patients so fatigued or weak that even the mildest form of exercise is not an option. Obviously, when there's a serious injury, an exercise program is going to have to be carefully tailored by the physician or physical therapist. But when it's possible, a time of being outdoors or gentle stretching/meditative exercise can be very beneficial as a stress reducer.

As a caregiver, you are under a burden of stress that can ruin your health. What's good for your patient is good for you, too. Thirty minutes of exercise a day is a great stress-buster. You don't have to do it all at once. If your patient is house-bound, you can take your exercise in short spurts throughout the day. The object is to be creative about the ways you work it into your schedule, and to make the exercise you choose something you enjoy doing.

Acupuncture can mitigate side effects. Ms. Herczog reported that she also used the eastern practice of acupuncture as a means of lessening the side effects of the chemo:

I had already been seeing an acupuncture/Chinese medicine doctor... she promptly put me on herbal pills, which she said would keep my blood-cell count up (white blood cells often are severely reduced by chemotherapy) and another to deal with the chemo side effects.

Coincidentally, right at this time, the American Medical Association gave its seal of approval to acupuncture for dealing with nausea from chemo.[10]

Dad, a World War II vet, openly declared that he was *not* a touchy-feely person. Alternative and complementary medicines, for him, were definitely a touchy-feely process. And yet, during his long illness and its debilitating treatments, he willingly went to an acupuncturist/herbalist, at the suggestions of his oncologist (who, in my opinion, was the epitome of a non-touchy-feely physician). I was surprised the doctor suggested it and even more surprised that Dad went. He did not maintain the practice for a prolonged period, but while he went and while his condition was at a somewhat stable point, he said he did get some relief from the side effects of the particular chemo he was taking.

Healing touch has been shown to be beneficial. There is a wide variety of healing touch techniques, almost all of them spiritually based. In some, there is a direct hands-on-the-patient approach to the technique. Others don't actually involve touching the patient but having the practitioner move their hands about two inches above the patient's body.

The ancient Japanese practice of Reiki is another example of a healing touch practice that can be helpful as a complementary addition to the medical treatments your loved one is receiving. Pronounced *ray-kee,* the word translates into universal life energy. This healing technique involves the laying on of hands to balance the subtle energies of the physical body, the emotions, and the mental and spiritual energy of the patient. In deciding on whether to use Reiki or another healing touch, it's important to understand the difference between the concepts of healing and cure, which I outlined in Lesson Five, "The Medical Team."

Consider how you might benefit from touch as well. What are you willing to do? There are the mini-massages that come with manicures or pedicures, chair massages like the ones you can get in airports. Of course, there are full massages of all kinds to be found in health spas. This is another one of those practices that's good for caregivers as well as patients.

Biofeedback, visualization, hypnosis, and meditation can be helpful techniques. We of Western culture have a tendency to get into our heads the belief that the best way to solve a problem is to reduce it to its component parts and fix the ones that are broken. It's the same mechanistic approach on which our medical practices are based. One of the problems with this idea is that it separates the totality of the self into two basic components—mind and body. The mind is seen as an entirely separate entity from the body, and the emotional and spiritual are generally not taken into account at all. Treatment in this system focuses on the mechanism that is the body, without input or participation from any other aspects of the self. The patient may not be best served by such a separation.

Techniques such as biofeedback, creative visualization, self-hypnosis, hypnosis, guided meditation, and meditation use the concept of altering our state of being, achieving a deeply-relaxed state in which the forces of the intellect and emotion can be engaged in the physical process of healing. In all of these techniques, a beneficial state of deep relaxation is involved. I believe that when we engage all of our faculties—

physical, mental, emotional, and spiritual—in the treatment, the results are going to be more positive than if we just let the body do the work in solitary confinement.

Ms. Herczog also began seeing a hypnotherapist:

> Alas, she does not wave a watch in front of my face and announce that I am getting sleeeepy. Rather, she maternally tucks me in and has me listen to wave sounds while she calmly tells me to relax and visualize. It doesn't take long before I'm out—napping or hypnotized, call it what you will. During this time [she] makes suggestions about, among other things, strengthening my immune system, keeping my attitude positive, and developing relaxation techniques to reduce discomfort. This is taped, and I take the tapes home to listen to at night. It is so soothing and comfortable that often, immediately post-chemo when I'm not feeling so great and listening to one of her tapes, I think I can't wait to go to Janet again so I can feel good.

In closing, Ms. Herczog noted of her acupuncture/herbalist and her hypnotherapist, "It's my doctors who are going to cure me, but these two women are going to help me feel better during the process."[11]

Journaling is a way to give expression to feelings. If you are looking for blessings in your time of darkness, certainly practices like meditation or self-hypnosis can be helpful. Keeping a daily journal is another practice that is crucial for me because I can express my thoughts and emotions, especially those feelings that I don't want to share with anyone else. I have used journaling intermittently during my life, but during my sister's illness, it became an absolute necessity.

Journaling requires a bit of discipline to set aside the time to put a pen onto a piece of paper and write something every day. The blessings to be found by the caregiver are well worth the effort. All the unworthy thoughts and feelings now have a place to go, and believe me, getting them out, even if you never look at them again, takes their harmful power away. Julia Cameron, author of *The Artist's Way: A Spiritual Path to Higher Creativity*, notes that her journaling puts her in contact with "an unexpected inner power ... the [journal is] a pathway to a strong and clear sense of self."[12] Journaling is a practice that benefits whoever uses it—patient or caregiver.

Spiritual practices can be beneficial. In an earlier discussion about shadow experiences, I indicated that I believe certain types of faith healing are not only *not* beneficial but are also potentially damaging. However, I want to be clear that there are spiritual practices that are of assistance to people with serious illnesses and injuries and to their caregivers as well. I want to briefly touch on the benefits of personal prayer, intercessory prayer, and similar intercessory healing practices.

As I mentioned in the discussion of meditation practices, invoking all of the self in the healing process, and especially the spiritual along with the physical, has been well documented as being beneficial in such work as Dr. Dale Matthews's *The Faith Factor: Proof of the Healing Power of Prayer*, Dr. Larry Dossey's *Healing Words: The Power of Prayer and the Practice of Medicine*, and *Prayer Is Good Medicine*, as well as recent studies at Dartmouth Medical Center and at Duke University's Center for the Study of Religion/Spirituality and Health and the university's Ischemia Monitoring Laboratory.

There are countless stories of people who have experienced physical relief after being the subject of concentrated prayer by others. Cyndy, a young woman from my church, was hospitalized for thirteen days as a result of complications from treatments for both breast and ovarian cancer. An additional surgery seemed imminent. She describes herself as lying in a bed "looking like a science project because [she] was hooked up to so many machines."

One night, she awoke and sat up in her bed, completely awake, alert, and calm. After about an hour, she felt drowsy, lay back down, and went to sleep. What she didn't know was that at that same time, the members of her Bible study group were engaged in concentrated intercessory prayer for her. The next day, a hospital technician stopped by and prayed with her briefly. "She was like an angel; she was in my room, prayed with me, and was quickly gone," Cyndy recalls. The X-rays taken the day following the angel visitation indicated that the intestinal blockage that had appeared to be developing had cleared. There would be no need for additional surgery.

Mary Susan Herczog reported a similar experience with a friend's Reiki group.

> One Sunday morning, after an unexpectedly bad Friday with severe intestinal pain and a Saturday spent recovering, I leaped out of bed feeling just fine. I noticed this particularly because the change seemed to come out of the blue. The next day, I learned that minutes before, my friend Christopher's Reiki II group had been focusing all their energies on me and my healing.[13]

Studies on the effect of prayer on a patient's physical condition show that three types of prayer—colloquial, or a conversation with God; meditative; and intercessory—are all beneficial in that they produce positive physiological changes in patients. Oddly, petitionary prayer—the type used in faith healing—and ritualistic prayer are not as consistently associated with beneficial results but instead show increased stress among patients.

What You Can Do

Like Mary Susan Herczog and her delight in chocolate, there are simple pleasures that you can provide to your loved ones that can ease their discomfort and lift their spirits.

- *A new look through a makeup party or makeover*—For women, especially if there are physical changes as a result of their condition, trying out a new look can be a necessity. The cancer center at our local hospital annually invites cancer patients and makeup specialists to a party so the women can learn techniques for making themselves look and feel as attractive as possible. For my sister, who went reluctantly, it was a major boost to her sense of well-being. If there's not an opportunity through a hospital or cancer center, you can take your loved one to the makeup counter at the local department store. Maybe now's the time to invite your loved one's closest friends to a cosmetics party in your home.

- *A hat and scarf party*—This can be adapted to whatever piece of clothing your loved one is going to need while dealing with treatment, but the most obvious example is for people who are losing their hair because of chemo treatments. Women are assumed to be most affected by hair loss, but men suffer from hair loss too. Have a party—a shower—and invite everyone to bring a hat or a large square scarf that can be tied turban-like around the patient's head. Men have a distinct advantage here in that it's socially acceptable for them to have a bald head, in the era of the bald celebrities and star athletes. If the bald look isn't for them, they might want to start a baseball cap collection. Choose hats that are soft so as to not irritate the tender, newly exposed scalp. For women, choose hats that can cover all of the head where their hair used to be. Some even come with fake bangs to further disguise the hair loss.

• *Flowers*—One thing that spouses, partners, and significant others can do for their loved ones is to bring flowers. Not just when they're in the hospital, but afterwards, when they're home, struggling through treatment and adjusting to a new lifestyle. My sister really, really did not want to receive flowers when she was hospitalized. "It makes me think of funerals," she would grouse. My brother-in-law heard what she said but also understood that flowers can bring blessings too, so he arranged to have a fresh bouquet delivered to their home once a week when she wasn't hospitalized. She looked forward to the arrivals of the flowers and would rearrange them, if she wasn't too ill. They were a source of pride, a physical manifestation of Chuck's love for her, and they cheered her up beyond the value of a few stems with blossoms on the ends. Chuck had flower arrangements delivered from the local florist, but it's not necessary to go to that expense. A branch from one of your flowering fruit trees, a nosegay of flowers from your garden, or a single rose with a bit of fern will do as much for your loved one as the big, beautiful bouquet from the florist.

• *A manicure/pedicure*—Whether you're a man or woman, adult or child, having your nails done is one of life's important little pleasures. It can provide a boost beyond just the application of nail polish. Taking your loved ones to a salon may not be possible because of their condition. Can you arrange to have the manicurist come to the house or hospital room? Can you do the manicure yourself? I think part of the benefit is not just that hands and feet look nicer when it's done; it's the human touch that counts. Patients who are being constantly poked and prodded by medical people probably appreciate a soothing hand or foot massage more than the rest of us can imagine.

- *Massage*—If a hand or foot massage feels good, then your loved ones might really enjoy a therapeutic massage. This can be a tricky proposition if they've never had one before—it may seem invasively intimate. If they decline, let it go. But it can also be both soothing and deeply relaxing, both of which are beneficial. You can take them to a masseur or masseuse, have the massage come to them, or, if neither of those options is possible, learn some elementary massage techniques yourself. Facials that use warm face cloths and soothing lotions are also a way of providing the relaxing touch that patients find enjoyable. Again, it can be done professionally, or you can learn some elementary techniques and give the facial to your loved one yourself.

- *Aromatherapy*—This is not for everyone. People who dislike perfumes and incense may find this more irritating than helpful. The principle is that aromas from specific herbs and herb combinations can play a role in healing various minor illnesses or in altering emotional states. It is another way to soothe and relax patients and to provide them the means to a meditative state. Aromatherapy supplies—candles, oils, diffusers, or incense—can be found anywhere, from the nearest Asian herbalist to the local Walmart.

- *Candles*—Think of these as being aromatherapy lite. Sometimes homes where patients are confined to bed take on a distinctive sick room smell. Placing some lighted candles in the patient's room, as well as in the primary public rooms—hallway and living room usually—will alleviate this problem. Even at high noon, a few candles lend a warm atmosphere, as well as chase away the undesirable odors. Years after my sister's death, her husband, Chuck, still enjoys having a few candles lighted when he's at home because of the warm, pleasant atmosphere they provide.

• *Music*—Having some background music playing softly is another way to establish a soothing, healing atmosphere. This doesn't mean it has to be elevator music or vapid New Age air pudding music. What do your patients like to hear? Depending on their taste and circumstances, it could be anything from Mozart to Mötley Crüe. However, I'd save the hard rock for when your patients are doing some hard, physical work with a physical therapist and keep the Mozart or John Tesh on tap for times when relaxation and stress reduction are the goal. My sister really enjoyed Broadway show recordings and movie sound tracks, especially the one from *Emma*, as well as New Age recordings that combined piano music with sounds from nature, so that's what we played for her. In addition, for myself, I created a tape that I called comfort music, which included some sacred choral favorites, some jazz piano, and a couple of favorite Broadway tunes. That tape lived in my car for eighteen months during MaryKay's illness and after her death. I put it away eventually, but it came back out, to live in my car sound system again with Dad's final illness. I still use it now in times of stress.

- *Books, DVDs, and books on tape*—If your patients' activities are restricted because of their condition, books and DVDs or videos can be an outlet for them. Like the music collection, this is the time to surround them with their favorites and to provide those books and movies that they've always meant to get to. Remember that some treatments and procedures, such as use of a heart-lung machine in surgery, cause problems with concentration, memory, or vision, so your loved ones may go through these more slowly, taking more time to back up and check the plot points than they normally would. If reading books is not an option because of vision or other physical problems, then books on tape can be a great gift.

- *Comfort foods*—Do you remember when you were a child and you fell down and banged your knees or caught a cold? What special foods did your mother make for you? For my sister and me, it was steamed white rice, buttered and mixed with sugar, cinnamon, and milk—a quick version of rice pudding. When I'm feeling crummy, guess what I want to have for dinner? That's right, Mom's rice dish. Comfort foods are exactly that, the foods that take us back to a time when we were being soothed. With your loved one facing a serious illness, now is the time to prepare those comfort foods. Obviously the warning here is that comfort foods are beneficial *as long as they are not forbidden for medical reasons.* When it's possible, taking the time to provide meatloaf, macaroni and cheese, tuna casserole, or chopped liver on fresh rye bread can be a great gift to your loved one.

- *Play and joy*—Laughter is a form of medicine that produces beneficial physical changes in the body—the release of chemical substances called endorphins—that just generally makes people feel better. In all the serious issues facing your loved ones, a sense of joy, the relief of laughter, and time for fun should be included with everything else that you're doing to help them. Board games or card games, if they are played in a non-competitive manner, can provide a time of laughter and fun. Comedies on DVD, video, or at the movies can be wonderful producers of laughter. Don't be afraid to be silly. The assignment is to find ways to invoke laughter and joy.

- *A place in the sun*—This is meant literally and figuratively to include all the little things you can do to provide physical comfort to your loved one. My sister suffered from chills quite a bit when she was going through chemo. I brought her the chaise lounge off my patio so she could lie in the warm sun on her deck. Do your loved ones suffer from tender feet or hands? Perhaps a soft pair of gloves or slippers would provide comfort. Egg crates made of foam, lamb's wool for irritated and sore elbows and knees when they're confined to bed; these are the types of things you can provide to give them a bit more physical comfort.

There are no deep secrets to any of this. Think about the physical comfort of your patients and ask yourself what you can to do make them feel better. Anything you or they come up with will be a blessing.

LESSON SEVEN:
THE PATIENT'S TEAM

January 29, 1998

I don't know this friend of Claudette's, but she's one of the many who, having heard about MK's recurrence, wants to do something to help. For the most part, that desire to help is merely frustrating for them—and for us—because there's so little anyone can do. They can't cure MaryKay, they can't come up with a better medical treatment, and they can't pick up her life and live it for her while she cycles out to heal. But they can—and do—bring in dinners, drive to doctors' appointments, do the shopping, and connect us to people like Dr. Hoda Anton-Culver and her epidemiology study at UC Irvine Cancer Center. Thanks to Claudette's friend, I was reassured after talking to this doctor about family tendencies and how they may—or may not—affect us, especially Diana (my daughter). I hope someday these good deeds will come back around to all of these people who have tried to help us when they need comfort or support.

J ust as there is a medical team of physicians and other medical professionals for the patient, the patient needs a support team too, one that is beyond the one or two people who support the patient in the medical realm. The good news is that it's fairly easy to create a team for the patient because people are going to offer to help when word of your loved one's medical condition gets out to the larger circle of neighbors, friends, and business colleagues. It's inevitable. Rabbi Kamin, in *The Path of the Soul,* writes that this response is inherent in human beings because it's part of our creative nature. When faced with the life-threatening condition of a loved one, we turn to our particular capability, be it cooking, gardening, or even simple conversation. We are blessed in serving them by being able to use our own creative abilities. "The results are subjective, personal, and, often enough, redeeming," he writes.[1]

As comforting as these offers of help are to both the patient and the volunteers, they can also be vexing because these can come in overwhelming numbers but with *under-whelming* results. Once the patient has moved through the diagnosis, has selected a medical team, and is in the routine of the treatments, some decisions need to be made about this second circle of support that's being offered.

There are really two tiers of support: the small group of intimates and a larger circle of volunteers. Both levels of caregiving are needed, and both constitute the patient's team. The inner circle—the A team—consists of the patient's closest circle of intimates, the people who are the longtime friends or neighbors with whom the patient shares a deep bond. They are spouses and life partners and family members—parents, siblings, or children.

Volunteers are the next tier, the B team that comprises the wider circle of friends and acquaintances whose lives intersect with the patient's and who care enough to want to do something to be supportive. The support of both the inner circle and the wider circle of volunteers is important to patients not just because of the service provided but because it can be helpful to them in terms of their ability to handle the stress of their medical condition. Dr. Dale A. Matthews, in *The Faith Factor*, notes:

> The importance of having a functioning social network increases in times of stress, such as illness and aging, when social support often includes not only emotional sustenance but also practical assistance, like rides to the doctor's office and help with strenuous household chores.[2]

Accepting Help

How, or if, others outside of this inner circle are allowed to help is, of course, up to the patients. That decision may be based on their physical condition. If they feel well, they may not want any additional help. My friend Cheryl didn't need much assistance when she was going through chemotherapy. The normal reaction of volunteers is to offer help with meals and running errands. But Cheryl had a mild reaction to her treatment that didn't prevent her from cooking and generally keeping her home and family functioning. However, as a college instructor, she did need help covering her classes while she was recovering from surgery, something that her colleagues were able to do for her.

Help from volunteers may also be declined when the patient or members of the inner circle are in denial. If patients are not in touch with the reality of their circumstance, they won't perceive they need help. For instance, they may insist they don't need help of any kind but end up hospitalized for malnutrition because they haven't been well enough to prepare meals. Sometimes the help is turned away not by the patients but by their spouses or other family members who are in their own denial of the patient's condition and need for help.

Valerie, a woman I met through a mutual friend, struggled through her final days of bone cancer because her mother and her adult daughter were in such deep denial of her pending death that they persistently insisted that Valerie didn't need any help. In their denial, they saw her as being just fine when she clearly was not fine at all.

Accepting offers of help are not always easy because of the patient's psychological makeup. It gets back to the problem of being perceived as needy or incapable of taking care of oneself. There is also an emotional issue for some people about being able to receive expressions of affection, which is what these offers of help are. A person who is used to being in the role of giving out the support doesn't always want to be on the receiving end of it, for a variety of complex reasons. All of these factors may affect the patient's decision in accepting or declining offers of help from volunteers.

How Can I Help?

Wanting to *do* something is such a natural response to learning someone we know is in a crisis situation. That's why the first question always is, "How can I help?" It is sometimes puzzling, then, that so little results, even when the patient may respond affirmatively—"Yes, please, I could use some help with meals or housework or errands." The list of areas where volunteers can be of service is as lengthy as the offers usually are plentiful. So then why does so little of benefit to the patient actually happen?

I believe there are a couple of reasons. The first and most common reason I've observed is that there's no defined plan for the volunteer to follow. They offer a meal. The offer is accepted. Now what? Without a specific meal to prepare—a date and time to deliver it—the offer is left in a free-floating state while both parties vaguely wonder why the other isn't providing what they need. On the patient's side, of course, the question is, "Where's the meal?" But the volunteer needs to know exactly what meal, what day and time, how much food, what's acceptable, and what can't—or won't—be eaten. Without that kind of information, the meal rarely materializes.

Another reason help isn't accepted is because it either isn't needed at that moment or the recipient can't figure out what help is needed. That was certainly my case when my sister was in treatment for the recurrence of her cancer. My friends all offered help to me, but I could not come up with something for them to do. I wasn't sick, though I was caring for my sister and running our business, which created a very high stress level, which my friends saw and wanted to help relieve. Rather than turn them down, I banked their offers by telling them I couldn't think of any help I needed *at the moment,* but I would appreciate being able to call on them for assistance at some point in the future.

That point came not long after my sister died. My husband and I had temporarily moved out of our house to do a remodel project—more stress—assuming it would take more than six months. It was done in a little more than three months, and we were going to move again just as I was dealing with funeral arrangements and the aftermath of MaryKay's death. To say the prospect of packing up and moving again was overwhelming would be a vast understatement, so I cashed in the banked offers of help.

One group of friends came on a Friday and cleaned up the construction mess in the kitchen, pantry, and bathrooms so I could move back in.

One dear friend lined the pantry shelves and kitchen cabinets with shelf paper. As it was self-adhesive shelf paper, the most difficult to work with, you can see that this was a gift of great magnitude.

The next day, eight more friends showed up with their trucks, SUVs, and vans. I supplied the boxes, shipping tape, stacks of old newspapers, snacks, soft drinks, and a lunch. They supplied the labor. Working together, we managed to get all of the items I didn't want the movers to touch packed up and moved the few blocks back to my newly-remodeled home. We finished in about six hours, setting the stage for the movers to come on Monday. It was a joy to share this arduous process with my friends, and I was relieved of a hugely stressful task.

The point I hope you caregivers will absorb is that you, like the patient, will be the subject of your friends' and family's concern. The offers of help will be made for the patient and for you too. Please do not turn these offers aside because you are not the patient. It's an easy trap to slip into—you're healthy, so why should you need or accept an offer of help? You need support just as much as the patient does. The offered meal, help with the housework, or even just a general offer of help are for you too. Think seriously about using them or banking them as I did.

Organizing Volunteers

When the patient and the inner circle are ready to accept help from volunteers, there are ways to create the structure that eases the process for patient and volunteers alike. Having someone who can coordinate the volunteers requires a bit of organizational skill, so that is the first volunteer position you should fill, assuming there's an administratively adept person who has volunteered. It's a key job when there are people outside the small inner circle who are offering to help. This position can be used to coordinate a whole range of volunteer activities such as meals, housework, yard work, errands, and child care. Or, depending on the patient's needs, it may be limited to just arranging for meals to be delivered.

Meals are probably one of the most important services volunteers can provide to both the patient and the caregiver. Obviously patients and their families are going to need to eat, so having meals provided is an important service. Food is probably more imbued with personal expression than any of the other services that volunteers can provide. The way we prepare food is truly an expression of who we are, and it reflects, in some ways, our feelings about the people for whom we prepare it. With that idea in mind, it is really important to have someone who can frame these meal gifts in a way that works well for the patient.

When my sister realized she could not fix meals for her husband and son due to her weakened condition, she started accepting the offers of meals, asking various people to bring dinners on specific nights. Because she was so ill and unable to give much in the way of direction to her friends, the results were often not good:

- Volunteers weren't always clear who was bringing dinner on which night, so sometimes no meals would materialize, and sometimes two would show up on the same night.

- The appropriateness of the dinners was sometimes questionable, since the volunteers didn't know what the food preferences of her family were. One volunteer brought a complete turkey dinner—in the middle of September—that would have fed a family of twelve. Another brought a scant few leftovers she found in her own refrigerator.

- Leftovers from these volunteer meals became a problem because there was no opportunity to eat them. They stacked up in the refrigerator until they spoiled and were thrown out. The huge turkey dinner, which the volunteer doubtlessly thought was a good idea specifically because it generated leftovers the family could eat, only created storage problems.

After a few weeks of these kinds of problems, my brother-in-law, Chuck, appointed a meal coordinator. Susie, a close friend and an excellent cook, took over coordinating the volunteers who wanted to bring in meals. She set a few easily-understood standards as to meal size and content and created a communications network for the meal volunteers so that she—and they—could communicate quickly and efficiently. It was a great gift to my sister and her family to know that dinners were no longer going to be a stress point.

As a member of her inner circle, I was also a meal volunteer, but with a difference—I brought the ingredients on Sunday nights and cooked the meal in her kitchen. The menu ran heavily to our family's favorite foods. By spending time in preparing and sharing the meal, MaryKay and I had ample time to visit, and there was also time for me to be with her husband and teenage son when we all sat down to dinner together. I would *not* recommend that all meal volunteers bring in the raw ingredients and cook in the patient's kitchen. That's a process more appropriate to family and the closest friends—the inner circle.

An example of another need for volunteers concerned my friend Archie in the final weeks of his struggle with prostate cancer. He was single and his adult children all lived out of state. The chemotherapy he was taking to control the tumors that were then in his bones had to be limited in duration because it posed a threat to his heart. When this medication—which had been keeping the tumors at bay—was withdrawn, Archie was in severe pain. The doctor prescribed a strong painkiller, but it left Archie in a foggy state, a danger to himself. Friends from church became aware of his predicament, and so we took turns sitting with Archie in his home, making meals, and keeping him out of danger until his children arrived a week later.

Depending on the patient's needs and lifestyle, there are a limitless number of ways in which offers of help can be put to use. One thought to keep in mind is the duration of the need. Is the patient's condition chronic, meaning that the inability to cook meals, clean house, do yard work, care for children, or whatever the need may be will be permanent? If so, it will change the way in which volunteers can be expected to provide help. If the need is short-term, due to a temporary disability, then use of volunteers will likewise be short-term. Some people prefer the long-term assignments and some the short-term assignments. Be sure that the patient and the volunteers are all clear as to the nature of the need and how it will be met.

Thanking Volunteers

Good manners dictate that we thank others when they give us something or provide help in some way. However, the necessity for thanking volunteers who are helping care for your loved one goes beyond being merely polite. As Rabbi Kamin notes, the volunteers are bringing gifts of their hearts in providing their particular service to your patient. And so the thank you needs to come from the heart of the recipient, not just from a set of rules in an etiquette book.

None of this needs to be elaborate, expensive, or time-consuming. A spoken thank you at the time the meal is delivered

or the groceries are brought home from the store can be meaningful if it's heartfelt—"I really appreciate what you're doing.
It makes me feel better to have friends like you helping me
out this way." A phone call from the patient to a volunteer to
express thanks also works. If the corps of volunteers is large or
they are providing a wide range of services over a long period
of time, there are other ways you and your loved one can offer
thanks to them:

- E-mail is an easy way of reaching a lot of people at one
  time, if the patient and volunteers have it. There are a
  number of electronic cards available online that can be
  mailed out to thank the volunteers for their help.

- Do the volunteers have something in common, such as
  being fellow employees of your loved one, or members of
  a club, civic organization, or church? You can make use
  of the institution's newsletter to offer thanks to them.

- Your loved ones may want to create their own newsletter, a photocopied piece they can mail out to their
  volunteers as a way of thanking all of them.

- If you live in a small town, perhaps the local radio station, cable outlet, or newspaper would allow your loved
  ones to make a PSA (public service announcement)
  in thanking the people who have been assisting them.

- Thank you notes are always appropriate, but the use
  of them will be limited by the patient's energy and
  resources. If there are just a few volunteers, then mailing a note or even an art postcard is a good way to say
  thanks for the help.

- If the patient recovers from the illness or injury, then
  gathering all of the volunteers for a party is certainly

a good way to say thank you while celebrating the patient's return to health. It doesn't need to be fancy or expensive—a hot dog roast in the local park is just as festive and says thanks just as well as a sit-down dinner at a local restaurant.

What You Can Do

Here are some ideas about how those offers of help can be put to use for your patient. The complexity of the need will vary from patient to patient and will change for each individual over time as his or her treatment and condition changes. The jobs are listed in categories of the help that patients may need.

- *Volunteers*—This is a job for someone with good organizational and people skills, to assist a patient whose needs cover a wide range. This person would be a captain of captains, making sure meals are being coordinated and that needs for help with housework, child care, errands, and medical appointments will be met. This person can do all the coordinating themselves or assign sub-coordinators in each area of need, depending on the complexity of the circumstances. This job would normally be done by patients, but if they are acutely ill or undergoing strenuous or debilitating treatments, then it's a better idea to have a non-patient handle this job. Ideally, it can be done by a member of the inner circle.

- *Meals*—This person is the one who sets up the corps of meal providers, arranges a communication system among them, schedules the meal deliveries, and also sets some standards for quality, quantity, and content.

Meals don't have to be gourmet or even made at home. What they need to be is appealing to both the patient and the family. There's nothing wrong with occasionally picking up a pizza from the local takeout, provided the patient's family likes to eat pizza. Keep in mind that just because you like anchovies, it doesn't necessarily follow that they will find anchovies a tasty treat. There also needs to be a plan for the leftovers. If there's no one in the home during the day to eat them, they just will clog the refrigerator until they spoil and need to be tossed out. Even when they know they're not going to eat them, patients and their families will store leftovers—like the complete turkey dinner— until they've turned into biology experiments, rather than put the leftovers immediately into the trash. It's not easy to throw out perfectly good food, especially when someone has prepared it for you. Cleaning out a refrigerator of fuzzy, green, and slimy food isn't fun either. It's a better idea to save on that particular form of labor by getting the meal providers to scale down the size of the meals so leftovers aren't a problem.

- *Medical Team*—This is the job outlined in Lesson Five, "The Medical Team." Another title might be advocate, scribe, or appointment buddy. This is the person who is the second set of eyes and ears during medical appointments. This person ideally would be very close to the patient because there is a deeply personal aspect to any medical appointment.

- *Calendar*—This was a job we discovered as my sister became so weak that she could not be left alone in her home. There were treatments and medical appointments that she needed to be driven to, and her son, an active teenager, had activities that he needed to be taken to. So we appointed a calendar coordinator whose job it was to ensure that someone was available to be with MaryKay during the day, to get her to the appropriate medical appointment, and to get her son to his various activities. An important ingredient in this process is the patient's input. MaryKay was always a part of the scheduling process, both to assure herself that all of the necessary bases were covered and also to retain a sense that she still had some control over her life.

- *Child Care*—Where there are children, there is always a need for help. It doesn't matter whether the children in question are toddlers or teenagers; helping with the kids is a great gift to the patient. This can include obvious things, like babysitting for younger children when their parent is hospitalized or unable to care for them, even if the parent is being cared for at home. Driving children to athletic practices and events, church group meetings, music lessons—the whole range of kids' activities—can be a great help. Children whose parents are ill are under a great deal of stress and can use lots of support, so having someone spend time with them in meaningful ways helps them as well as the patient. School performance can lag, so offering to help with schoolwork can be a great benefit. Taking a child shopping for school clothes or other needs is another way to support both the child and the patient. Where it is difficult to find a volunteer to provide this support, consider organizations such as Big Brothers/Big Sisters or the YMCA and similar groups that have mentors available for children. These long-term relationships with adults can be very beneficial if the parent is suffering from the long-term or chronic condition that limits his or her ability to be with his or her child.

- *Spouse Relief*—You who are the spouses or life partners of patients with life-threatening illnesses are under immense stress, trying to maintain your home and family while caring for your loved one. It's very important for your well-being to be relieved of the day-to-day pressure occasionally. In her book *On Death and Dying*, Dr. Elisabeth Kubler-Ross advocates that spouses be given a regular time off "by finding a helping hand for one evening a week during which time he can go bowling perhaps, enjoying himself without feelings of guilt and by letting off some steam which he can hardly do in the house of a very sick person." Tom, a longtime friend, took on the sole responsibility of caring for his wife, Beverly, during her final illness. Because he was retired, he believed he could devote himself full time to Beverly without need of relief. But Beverly knew the toll his constant care of her was taking and regularly asked him what he was doing to take care of himself. Tom got into the habit of taking an hour off in the early morning when she was asleep to take a walk and go to a nearby gym to work out briefly. Chuck, my brother-in-law, was urged strongly by my sister to maintain his routine of playing golf with a group of friends every Saturday morning. Staying with the patient while the spouse or life partner gets out to do something to relieve stress on a regular basis is a very important volunteer task.

- *Transportation*—When a patient is recovering from a serious injury or is in a weakened state from their illness, getting to appointments or running normal errands can become a major problem. Providing transportation, whether it's driving patients or assisting them with public transit, is a significant part of the help they need. I divide my time between suburban Southern California and rural Colorado where the car is king and public transit is a difficult way to travel. In places where cars are a necessity, the assistance is to drive patients to their various appointments. For those who live in urban areas with well-developed train and bus systems, the assistance may be in getting them onto a train or bus and riding with them to the appointment or arranging for and riding along in a taxi.

- *Errands*—The daily rounds of marketing, picking up medications from the pharmacy, and bringing home medical equipment—the thousands of little errands that we all run—are another significant need for patients who are in a weakened state. Having someone take care of these duties when they cannot is another important way to help. Like meals, the items bought at a grocery store are very personal to individuals. If they want peanut butter, what kind do they like—natural or homogenized, chunky or smooth? The volunteers who take on this job need to approach their duties almost as if they were hunting treasure, seeking out the exact items requested by the patient. And both patient and volunteer need an extra dose of flexibility because it won't come out right every time. Sometimes the patient is going to have to be content with chunky peanut butter when they prefer smooth. What counts is the sincerity of the effort to find the smooth peanut butter, not necessarily whether it comes home from the market.

- *House Work*—Let's face it, this is not high on anyone's list of favorite activities, but it is a great gift to have a clean home, clean clothes, or a mown lawn and weeded flower beds. Any home requires a lot of effort, and when the family is focused on caring for an ailing member, especially if the ill person is one who does the housework, laundry, or yard work, then those functions are among the first to be ignored in favor of caregiving. I've done yard work for a church friend who suffered major injuries in a skiing accident. His wife noted that he would sit in his wheelchair staring out at their yard, clearly frustrated because he couldn't work in the garden he enjoyed so much before the accident. While these jobs aren't necessarily fun, think of them as being great stress relievers for patients and their families.

- *Job Support*—This is dependent on the patient's job or volunteer position being of a type that others could fill in. Recall the story of my friend Cheryl, the college instructor whose fellow faculty members taught her classes for a short period while she recovered from surgery. Another friend who was a host at our local ski area was sidelined with pulmonary embolisms. The other hosts took his shifts so he would not lose his ski privileges while he was hospitalized and recovering at home.

- *Hospital Support*—This is an idea that often is overlooked during a medical crisis but which means so much to patients' families. Ask for support while your loved ones are hospitalized. It can be something as simple as having someone bring you a homemade sandwich and something to drink while you're awaiting the outcome of a surgery or standing by while your loved ones are in intensive care. One friend was on twenty-four-hour watch at the hospital while her youngest daughter was recovering from surgery following a riding accident. Another friend made a picnic lunch and took it to the stressed-out mother who had been subsisting on hospital cafeteria and vending machine food. Years later, the recipient still recalls how loved and supported that simple gesture made her feel. While I was waiting for my sister to recover from brain surgery, my stepmother, Claudette, showed up in the intensive care waiting room one day with the best tasting smoothie I've ever had. It's these personal touches that can mean so much during a crisis. Small can be awfully big, depending on one's perspective.

- *Card Campaign*—This is a job for someone who can be very organized and who has access to a mailing list of your loved one's friends and family members. It can be used to support the patient, the caregiver, or both. One of my sorority sisters organized a card-mailing campaign for two others—Cindy, who was dealing with radical treatments for breast cancer, and Betsy, whose husband, Mike, was struggling to overcome a crippling injury from a car accident. Jan, the woman who put this project together, sent a group of us four postcards and a Valentine's card—it was a silly child's valentine, and we used them because it was that time of year; you can use your imagination to expand this idea. The point was to write a note on the postcard and mail one a week. The valentine was the big finish. We were cautioned: "Do not say get well. They are both in for a long haul, and they need to hear from you about your life or just a note that tells a joke or tells them you are thinking of them." For both of these women, the impact of receiving this deluge of postcards and valentines was immensely strengthening.

- *Communications Network*—Communication is so important that I saved it for last. Even if the corps of volunteers is a handful of people, efficient and effective communication is still hugely important. Everyone involved needs to be kept apprised of the patient's condition, to the extent the patient is comfortable in sharing that information. Additionally, the volunteers need to be able to communicate among themselves when schedules need to be changed.

There are a couple of ways to set up these communications networks. In my opinion, the best is a sort of cluster system, in which one person has the responsibility of calling three or four others, and, if necessary, those three or four call an additional group of three or four. Another way, which seems simpler but which I don't feel works as well, is a phone tree. A phone tree is a lineal system for providing communication. Each person calls the next person in line until the last person is reached. Then the last in line calls the person who initiated the call so that it's clear the whole tree has been reached. The problem is that if one person on this line isn't contacted or doesn't contact the next person, the people below them are left out of the loop.

In our electronic age, e-mail can be a great assist, but effective use of this system depends on everyone involved checking their mail on a regular basis. I offer this explanation of groups for those of you who are new to e-mail or not fully versed in how it works. Within the address book of whatever e-mail system you use, there is a way of creating a group. You give the group a name—such as "meal volunteers"—and then add the appropriate names and e-mail addresses of the individuals who are members of that group. When you want to send a note to the group, instead of addressing the e-mail to each group member or copying each of the group members individually, you merely type in the group name on the address line and your note will be sent to everyone you've identified as being a group member. It's fast and therefore efficient. But it depends on the willingness of all of the volunteers to incorporate regular use of e-mail into their communication system.

And don't forget patient-based Web sites such as www.caringbridge.com and www.carepages.com, along with Facebook as another electronic means of communicating with—and thanking—a large number of people.

- *Thanking Volunteers*—If communication in general is important, then communicating gratitude to the volunteers is supremely important. Whether this is done by the patient—which would be ideal—or by the immediate family, I believe that thanking people often is the most important gift patients can offer to their volunteers. It is not possible, in my opinion, to thank volunteers too often. Volunteers are motivated by their love for the patient and the patient's family, but they should not be expected to provide their support in a vacuum. They are providing blessings in the time of darkness by their presence and support. A heartfelt expression of thanks is also a blessing. It's a means by which the patients or their families can return the blessing to the volunteers.

- *Other Ideas*—This is a place where you can become as creative as you like in expressing and providing support for the patient. One way to support patients is by supporting research in their disease or condition. My husband, Paul, makes it a point to run in the Race for the Cure, an event held in several cities across the country to support the Komen Breast Cancer Foundation. A dear friend, Nanette, specifically enrolled in the initial Avon Three Day, a seventy-five-mile walk from Santa Barbara to Malibu, on behalf of my sister. I still get tears in my eyes remembering the evening I drove MaryKay to the triumphal finish of that event. MK was in her wheelchair, and somehow Nan found her in a huge crowd. What a gift to MaryKay! When my friend Betsy suffered a brain injury and didn't have health insurance, many, many friends staged fund-raising events to help her. College friend Mike was still recovering from a spinal injury when he participated in a fund-raiser for other similarly injured people, and his friends supported him with their contributions to the cause. The help that can be offered here is unlimited. What creative ideas can you come up with?

LESSON EIGHT:
BEING WITH THE PATIENT

April 10, 1999

I am so immersed in my busy-thing that I'm finding it difficult to let go of this stuff (houses, work, church, etc.). There are hundreds of things—no joke—I could do today: get plants for the front area in Jasmine Creek, do some yard work at Heliotrope House, clean up my home office, do the laundry, and on and on 'til midnight, at least. I'm really struggling to let go of *all* of it so that I can go over to her house, hang out, and be with her. No rushing off to pick fabrics, or supervise painters, or buy groceries, or fix dinner, or anything else. Just go over there and be there for as long as she and I need.

There are no secrets about being with patients—your loved ones—other than just that: *Be* with them. If there's a skill to be learned, it is of being, not of doing. By that I mean that when you spend time with your loved ones, do it on their terms, not on yours. Suspend *your* list of things that you want to say or do and come to the patients with nothing more on your agenda than to meet them where *they* are. Most often, being with them means listening to them and letting them have the safety and space to communicate what's important to them, as Dr. Siddall described in active listening. Dr. Kubler-Ross reminds us to let them set the tone since their condition has established the agenda. Sometimes being with them will mean *not* talking but sitting together in silence, very much a shift from doing to being.

Sharing time with your patients definitely will require you to let go of your need or desire to control their state of being, to *not* try to manage how they are in their illness or injury. It's not always easy to achieve this state of being when both of you are facing life and death questions.

As human beings, we tend to want to take big actions in the face of big challenges. The problem is that activity—doing instead of being—becomes a distraction that shuts off the opportunities to look at and talk about the things that are most important. Finding these inner treasures is one of the great blessings of your time together with the patient. It would be a shame to waste the opportunity by being so consumed with action plans that there is no space for the quiet moments of contemplation and deeper communication.

Psychiatrist M. Scott Peck says that the ability to suspend our action plans and truly be with someone who is suffering provides a form of redemption. In his book, *Denial of the Soul: Spiritual and Medical Perspectives on Euthanasia and Mortality,* he notes that:

> When a person bears the emotional pain of others in such a manner...others are in some way healed or redeemed as a result...The only truly loving thing I can do in this situation is to be willing to share your pain...and to say with genuine feeling, "God, I'm sorry. It must be awful for you. Can I sit here with you for a while, or would you rather be alone?"[1]

Valerie, the woman who was dying of bone cancer whom I wrote about in the last chapter, made a twenty-five-hundred-mile trip to visit a friend because she needed someone who could just *be* in the face of her imminent death. You may recall Valerie's mother and adult daughter could not accept that she was dying of bone cancer and insisted, right up to the end, that she was just fine. Their denial made it impossible for Valerie to talk about her feelings. As a result, she dragged herself across the country to a friend who provided the one thing she desperately needed—a willingness to suspend the need for action and simply listen to Valerie talk about her illness and her coming death. Meanwhile, back at home, Valerie's daughter was frantically seeking out *the* faith healer who could cure her mother. But Valerie didn't need an encounter with a faith healer; she needed those closest to her to be able to listen to her.

By now, you've noticed the importance of communication is a theme that's been emphasized in many of these lessons. Allowing for the flow of information between all involved—the patient, the medical team, the patient's team, and other family members, friends, and volunteers—is crucial, in my opinion. It is equally important that patients are allowed to share their feelings with the members of their inner circle, their caregivers. And so it is that in looking at ways to spend meaningful time with the patient, communication is once again a necessity. The fundamental need of your patients, beyond their medical circumstance, is to be able to talk to friends and family about what's happening to them. This is a basic need that we all have, and it's especially acute in a time like this.

The importance of this kind of sharing was brought home recently when I served on a jury that tried a man who had driven his car into a preschool playground, killing two children and injuring four more and a young female teacher. The young teacher testified at length about the horrible incident. She was composed, though emotional, in recounting her ordeal. But she completely broke down in pain-filled sobs when she related that she'd been forced to seek therapy after the incident because "no one [at the school] will let me talk about it." Your loved ones are no different from this traumatized young woman—they deeply need to be able to talk about their experience and their feelings.

When people like you, who are close to the patient, can provide this much-needed communications link, it can become the lifeline that keeps the patient grounded at times of extreme stress. Lorna Reed, a member of the board of trustees of the University of Southern California and a board member of the USC/Norris Cancer Hospital, is also a breast cancer survivor. In the *Winter* 1999/2000 *Cancer Report,* she noted that the worst part of having a life-threatening disease is the unknown and that it is extremely important that patients are able to talk about their feelings and fears.

Linda Quigley, one of the coauthors of *Speak the Language of Healing,* talks about the two women—one a close friend, the other her therapist—who served as her lifeline, beginning with the moments immediately preceding her mastectomy: "I needed them to save my life, for that day and days and months to come; they did, with so much love and acceptance that even now when I think of it the tears come in a hot flood."[2]

Ms. Quigley, an extremely independent and capable woman who is a Pulitzer Prize-winning journalist, was overwhelmed with the details necessitated by her new medical condition. She needed her friends to provide assurance that her concerns were manageable. "Did you get a room at the lodge for my parents? Are you sure someone is taking care of my cat? Am I going to get through this?"[3] Clearly the presence of her friends who listened and offered reassurance where they could made a huge difference in the way in which Ms. Quigley coped with her cancer and its treatment.

Quality time that you spend with your patients is based on this fundamental idea of allowing them to communicate their feelings and for you to share yours with them in a constructive way. The necessity of engaging in this deep level of communication goes beyond a simple sort of release valve function, the blowing off of emotional steam. The process in which both you and your patients are caught up is a life-changing one because it is a life-threatening one. When you allow your loved ones to talk about what is happening to them—physically, emotionally, and spiritually—you are providing blessings to them in this process of change by being their witness.

Physician and therapist Rachel Remens writes of this need to have our pain, hurt, hope, and fear validated by witnesses. In her book, *Kitchen Table Wisdom: Stories That Heal,* she reflects on how people with serious illnesses can feel terribly lonely and isolated by their medical condition. "I suspect that this sense of aloneness may even undermine the will to live. When we feel the support of others, many of us can face the unknown with greater strength."[4] She goes on to add later, "The places in which we are seen and heard are holy places. They remind us of our value as human beings. They give us the strength to go on. Eventually they may even help us to transform our pain into wisdom."[5]

I remember one brief conversation with my sister in which she talked about her death. She had stopped receiving treatment and was under the care of hospice. One afternoon she said she was really disappointed that she wasn't going to reach age fifty-three. "Why is that?" I asked. She was able to talk about all the hopes, plans, and dreams that she now had to acknowledge would go unfulfilled, especially her desire to watch her son grow into manhood. It was very painful to listen to, and I would have rather been just about anywhere else. But I also knew I was her witness and that my job in that moment was to hear her release her expectations of the future and accept that she would soon die.

I had a similar experience with my dad when he was in hospice care at the end of his life, only in his case I felt I was being called upon to witness the support, care, and nurture that he'd provided me throughout my life. "You're going to be okay, aren't you?" he asked me.

I reassured him that he'd done a great job in raising me and teaching me the family business so that I could become financially successful. "I'll be fine thanks to you," I told him. "I'll miss you terribly, but I'll be fine."

Isolation

The converse of this need is equally true—patients can feel a crippling sense of abandonment if they don't have someone with whom they can talk about what they are going through. Henri Nouwen, a writer on Christian spirituality, noted that "the roots of loneliness are very deep ... they find their food in the suspicion that there is no one who cares and offers love without conditions, and no place where we can be vulnerable without being used."[6]

Rabbi Ben Kamin in *Path of the Soul* relates the story of a woman, Emma, who was undergoing cancer treatment. Once an avid tennis player, she was forced by her illness and treatment to give up her regular weekly tennis game, and unfortunately her tennis friends didn't maintain their friendship once she stopped playing.

"There are days," Emma reported, "when I barely think about having cancer...life has changed for me since I was diagnosed. My tennis group still doesn't contact me. I was disappointed that twenty years with the same group of people meant so little to them."[7]

Emma earlier had suggested to Rabbi Kamin, "If you want to be a good friend to a cancer patient, listen. As a friend of a cancer patient, you should try to understand her feelings."[8] The same can be said of being a friend to anyone with any other serious illness or life-altering injury.

For all of the members of my family who struggled with life-threatening diseases—my mother, my sister, my father, my grandmother, and my mother-in-law—isolation was a real problem. Each one of these people, prior to the onset of their disease, had a large and seemingly close circle of friends. But as the disease progressed—and the threat to their lives grew more real—many of the friends dropped away, which left unhealed wounds. And there was no opportunity for reconciliation since the friends stayed away.

It's a phenomenon that I've pondered over the years, and I believe the answer to the withdrawal of some people during a medical crisis has to do with the missing friends' unresolved attitudes about death. When someone is dealing with a life-threatening circumstance, people who haven't confronted the issue of mortality—out of our inborn fear of death—are not going to want to encounter this issue as a friend or loved one struggles in that very arena. Instead, they will find excuses to stay away, some hating themselves for it, others unaware of their own transparency, and most feeling some degree of guilt.

If we, as caregivers, haven't confronted the issue of death in general, and our own deaths in particular, then we will face the same dilemma in being with our loved one who has a life-threatening or terminal illness. We'll become like the members of Emma's tennis group or some of my family's friends, and rather than face a loved one who may be coming to the end of life, we'll choose to stay away. Or we'll be like Valerie's family. Their denial also left Valerie in isolation, robbing her of the opportunity to talk about her feelings with those closest to her as she approached the end of her life.

The blessing of being a caregiver to someone who is seriously ill or injured is that we have an opportunity to examine our own feelings about the very human condition of death and of the meaning of the cycle of birth, life, and death. In the foreword of *Speak the Language of Healing,* physician and psychotherapist Jean Shinoda Bolen writes that "each of us gets our share and kind of suffering as an inevitable part of being human: what happens in us as a result makes all the difference to the psyche."[9]

We can't help but grow emotionally and spiritually when we begin to understand our place in the cycle of life. And that growth can only free us of our inhibitions about talking about these issues with our loved ones when they are facing such issues in a very real, physical way through suffering with their illness or injury. My stepsister, Carla, and her husband, Chris, made a point of visiting Dad in his last few difficult days. I found Chris at Dad's bedside one evening, just sitting with Dad as he slept. When he got up to leave, he promised my sleeping father that he'd be back again the next day. And he showed up as promised. That was a real gift of presence in the face of impending death.

Dr. Kubler-Ross, in *On Death and Dying,* notes that the topic of mortality isn't an everyday agenda item for the seriously ill. They have times they want to talk about it and times when they don't:

Patients are no different from the rest of us in that we have our moments when we feel like talking about what burdens us and times when we wish to think about more cheerful things, no matter how real or unrealistic they are. As long as the patient knows that we will take the extra time when *he* feels like talking, when we are able to perceive his cues, we will witness that the majority of patients wish to share their concerns with another human being and react with relief and more hope to such dialogues.[10]

Letting the Patient Set the Agenda

Dr. David Beadles is a Methodist minister who became a volunteer chaplain for his local hospice organization after he retired. He has a three-part standard for being with patients:

1. Let them talk.

2. Listen.

3. You can't fix it; just listen.

Dr. Beadles emphasizes the importance of letting your patients set the agenda. When they want to talk about issues, such as spiritual concerns, then you need to be willing to let them. And likewise, when that topic's not on the table, you need to be okay with that too.

For me, the absence of this important kind of conversation with my sister was troubling because I was *so* ready to talk about it. But discussions of mortality were nonexistent with my sister in the months immediately following the diagnosis of the recurrence of her cancer. I was working on my understanding of her mortality—and mine—and what that meant in terms of my faith in God. Because we were so close, it seemed natural that we would talk about these things, but she wasn't interested—

at all. In her unwillingness to talk about the meaning of her life and pending death, I learned an extremely important lesson about being with a patient—to simply be. As Henri Nouwen notes, "How simple a truth, but how hard to live! Being is more important than doing," or in my case, talking.[11]

Learning to be meant letting my sister decide what we'd talk about—or even if we'd talk—whenever we were together. Did she want to talk or remain silent? If she chose silence, I learned to sit in silence with her. If she didn't want to talk about herself but wanted to know what was going on at the office, I talked about the business. If she was dealing with an emotion like anger or sadness, my job was *not* to talk her out of it but to validate it—"Yeah, I can see why you'd feel that way." There were times when she was in mind-stretching denial. I learned to not *fix* her unrealistic perceptions but simply to let her express them.

Let me assure you that *none* of this was easy. I struggled with all of it, and it was only as she was diagnosed as being terminal that I could truly begin to incorporate these lessons into my life and into the way in which I interacted with her. Prior to that time, I wanted very much to have deep and meaningful discussions about life, death, and God with her, but when I brought them up, she let me know she didn't want to go there. Sometimes it was direct, as in the time she said, "You know, Joanne, sometimes you really overdo the God thing." Sometimes it was more indirect, by not responding to my opening remark and changing the subject.

Each of your patients is going to be different in the way in which they need to discuss their condition and their feelings. Cindy, a friend who was diagnosed with a very advanced stage of breast cancer shortly before my sister's death, had deep emotional struggles as she went through a very physically demanding series of treatments. Three of us who had been close friends in college decided it would be a good idea to get together with her on a regular basis. Cindy was clear about her needs and might say to us in advance of our getting together, "I'm feeling emotionally fragile today; let's not talk about it." It was easy to honor her request, and it was a relief that she could be direct with us about her needs because it saved us from having to guess which topics were taboo.

Cheryl, another college friend, needed an outlet to talk about her physical condition as she went through the process of treatment for her breast cancer, so she and I connected in phone conversations, mostly to share her joy at reaching the end of chemo or the steps in reconstructing her breast. Whatever the disease or condition and the anticipated outcome, the task of the caregiver is simply to endeavor always to remain open and accepting of the level of communication the patient needs at the time. The patient, your loved one, will be your guide.

Another aspect of the *being* that I learned from the illnesses of both my sister and father is the lesson of patience. Learning patience was learning to let her—and later him—set the tone for our time together. It was in being with her on her terms that allowed her to ultimately open up to the discussions about her life and death that I so wanted to have with her. My discussion with my sister came on her time, not mine, and in learning to wait for that, I learned an important lesson that applies to life in general—things happen when they are supposed to, not before. And they happen whether or not I've forced a conversation that my sister, or father, or anyone else, wasn't ready for. In Dad's case, that conversation occurred in an unexpected way, with his expressed concern over my future. With MaryKay, it happened in a way that we were able to have a full reconciliation and healing.

A Variety of Lessons

An important point to keep in mind during these times is that we can't predict what the lessons will be, how they will come to us, or what we'll learn. For instance, Dr. Kubler-Ross, writing in her latest book *Life Lessons,* notes that the lessons of patience for the caregivers are sometimes disguised and subtle and sometimes big with diseases such as Alzheimer's.[12] She goes on to note that we don't always get what we want. "You may want something right now but may not get it for a while, if ever. You will, however, always get what you need, even if it does not fit into your mental picture."

The lessons about simply being with a patient can include more than discussions of mortality and faith. Ané de Nio is the dear family friend who became MaryKay's companion for nearly six months and then again was with her in the weeks immediately preceding her death. Ané said she learned the same lesson on a seemingly much more trivial topic—shopping. Ané is, by her own admission, a very thrifty woman. MK, on the other hand, was a woman who took great joy in shopping. When they would make the rounds of department stores and shops, Ané was appalled at what she considered MaryKay's wasteful spending habits. At first, she tried to talk her out of some of her purchases, but like my attempts to discuss mortality, MK wasn't to be deterred. The tension over the issue was threatening to end their time together until Ané made the decision to let go of her attempt to control MaryKay's way of being.

"I learned to let go of my prejudices about someone else's behavior," she told me later. "And in doing that, in making room for them to be who they are, I could also release my need to control their behavior."

That was a big lesson, and learning it, Ané says, was a major blessing in her life because she now is able to carry it into her relationships with other people.

This idea of being with patients on their terms has some tricky aspects to it. One is the problem of optimism, which calls for a careful balance between realistic expectations and the will of your patients to struggle against their condition. We all recognize that people who look at their illness or injury as something to be overcome by them will probably experience as positive an outcome as possible, compared to those who give up and don't actively engage in their own recovery.

I've known two men—Rog, a business colleague, and Mike, a college friend—who both suffered potentially crippling spinal injuries. Both men simply refused to accept the medical prognosis that they would spend the rest of their lives in wheelchairs. Rog now walks, assisted by canes, and plays golf. Mike also walks with assistance. Neither man would be in the condition they are in now had they not possessed and marshaled a strong sense that they could overcome their injuries. A strong sense of optimism and a drive to improve impelled and inspired them both through the long and grueling recovery process.

One reason that sense of optimism and determination served Rog and Mike was that it was shared by their inner circles, the family and friends closest to them who supported them in their hard work. The key to the success of these patients and their teams was a balance in attitude between optimism about what could be achieved on the one hand and medical reality on the other. The balance Rog and Mike created makes an interesting contrast to the story of Valerie, where there was such imbalance between the patient and the false optimism held by her inner circle. Dr. Kubler-Ross notes that there needs to be a willingness of those closest to the patient to not be falsely optimistic, as Valerie's mother and daughter were. False optimism denies patients their reality, Dr. Kubler-Ross points out, and that is another way of shutting down communication—of leaving patients feeling isolated—because the people closest to them aren't able to see the truth of their circumstances.

The rule of thumb comes back to letting your loved ones set the agenda—letting go of your prejudices about behavior, letting go of your ideas of how they should be, and coming to your patients with patience, willing to see their circumstances through their eyes. You don't have to buy into what they may be feeling or doing, be it wild-eyed and unrealistic optimism or the passiveness of deep depression, but you don't have to change them either. Be willing to extend sympathy and accept them, wherever and however they are.

May I suggest caution, however, in the extent to which you assume you can offer acceptance and sympathy. There's a big difference between acceptance/sympathy and truly understanding their experience. That's what empathy is, and what it means is that while I could see my sister's struggle and suffering, I wasn't living it, so my understanding of it stopped short of her experience of it. Only someone else who's had a similar experience can truly empathize or share your loved one's feelings. I was introduced to this idea rather gently by my sister one day when I was telling her I knew how she felt.

"Actually, you don't," she said quietly. "Only someone's who's been through this can understand."

You can see what your loved ones are going through, you can commiserate with them about their pain and discomfort ("This must be really hard."), but you cannot truly share their experience, which is what empathy is. Only someone who's had the same illness and treatment, or injury, can truly empathize with them.

Healing

In the midst of your loved one's medical crisis, there are opportunities for significant blessings for you both in the form of healing, not necessarily of physical ailments but of ailments of the psyche and spirit. If you can see the potential for this coming to wholeness through reconciliation of broken relationships, it will be a bright light in your dark time.

MaryKay and I, for all of our closeness and love for each other, had wounds that we'd both suffered and inflicted on each other. As her physical condition deteriorated, we were able to find renewed emotional strength in healing those old hurts. It didn't involve a long list of here's what you did to me that hurt me. Instead, she simply said to me one day, "I'm sorry for all the times I let you down." It was a deeply moving moment for both of us because it opened the door to my forgiveness and for me to ask her forgiveness for all the times I'd hurt her. There were plenty of tears and hugs and a deep, quiet joy for each of us. And this instance allowed us a few more similar conversations of reconciliation of these old wounds.

In the wonderful book *Tuesdays with Morrie,* Professor Morrie Schwartz, who is suffering from Lou Gehrig's disease, philosophizes on the necessity to reflect on this aspect of our lives:

> "Mitch," he said, "the culture doesn't encourage you to think about such things until you're about to die. We're so wrapped up with egotistical things, career, family, having enough money ... we're involved in trillions of little acts just to keep going. So we don't get into the habit of standing back and looking at our lives and saying, 'Is this all? Is this all I want? Is something missing?'"[13]

Later, in their long-running conversations, Morrie tells author Mitch Albom:

"Forgive yourself before you die. Then forgive others."[14]

"[Forgive] ourselves?"

"Yes. For all the things we didn't do. All the things we should have done. You can't get stuck on the regrets of what should have happened. That doesn't help you when you get to where I am."[15]

I believe that the healing from this kind of reconciliation occurs in three ways. It can happen in all three categories, or it can be achieved in only one or two ways. But whether it's all or one, each part serves the purpose of providing emotional and spiritual wholeness to whoever is engaging in these healing processes:

- *Acknowledging of the wounds*—This doesn't need to be a detailed list, as was the case with my sister and me. For us, it was simply a statement about all the times we'd let each other down or hurt one another. And still, even something that brief could provide the acknowledgement that we each needed. These brief but intense moments of reconciliation allowed each of us to acknowledge the other as a whole human being, both as wounded and wounder. They were times of being seen for who we truly were by the other. It is a great gift to have a loved one recognize what happened earlier—be it days, months, or years earlier—because in doing that, they are validating who you are through that earlier experience.

- *Reconciliation*—I look at this process as the wiping clean of life's slate. Carrying around our wounds and our anger over them is hard work. One opportunity everyone who's facing life-threatening circumstances has is to lighten their load by cleaning off the slate where we keep track of these offenses against us. You don't have to be at death's doorstep to learn that it's not only possible, it's a good thing to offer forgiveness to someone who's harmed you and to reconcile old enmities. This is a tricky subject because most of the world's great faiths teach us, in some way, that we must unconditionally forgive those who have wronged us. I believe that we're required to forgive those who acknowledge the wrong that they've done. It takes a big soul—a whole lot of growth for most of us—to additionally reconcile with, or at least accept and forgive, those who have wounded us and who haven't asked forgiveness.

- *Releasing regrets*—We all carry a list of should-haves and could-haves with us, the things in our lives we never got to or decided not to get to. "I could have gone to law school if I'd studied harder and partied less in college." "I should have apologized to Aunt Edna for that spat we had five years ago. Now she's dead, and I can't tell her I'm sorry." "I should never have married so-and-so. Look how (he or she) wrecked my life." The list is endless. Like forgiveness of others, this is about forgiving yourself. The gift of healing is that in facing issues of life and death you or your loved one now have a larger, deeper backdrop against which the items on this list of regrets can seem pretty puny. And in seeing the regrets in this context, you are free to release them, forgiving yourself in the process.

Spiritual Issues

My struggle to learn to not force my need to discuss my faith on my sister when she was clearly unresponsive is one that many of you will go through in some degree. Spiritual concerns are obvious issues at a time when your loved one is facing a life-threatening condition, and so the lesson of simply being—and being patient—comes to the forefront.

You may be fortunate to have shared spiritual beliefs with your loved ones, and conversation about faith, life, and death will flow easily and effortlessly. On the other hand, you may not share their belief system—nor they yours—and so there can be times of awkwardness and discomfort as you try to honor their spiritual needs or practices. Or you may be like me and want to offer your reassurances about God's presence in the process and be rebuffed. It can be a delicate balancing act when you don't share the same faith or even the same *degree* of faith. But the lack of a shared spiritual belief system doesn't need to preclude conversation about these topics, providing no one feels compelled to convert the other to their point of view. It is indeed a delicate time of balancing the need to communicate with personal boundaries.

The onset of a serious illness or a disabling injury inevitably leads to a whole series of unanswerable questions about what divine act has caused the condition—the mysterious *why*. The implications of the question are enormous: Was it an act of the mindless mechanics of an impersonal universe? Did God decide to give it to your loved one, and if so why? Was it the result of some sinful act? Is God testing him or her—or perhaps you? Is there a spiritual or life lesson that God wants to teach either of you? Is it a Job-like test? Is it karma for a sin of omission or commission from another life? What happens if my loved one dies? Is death the end, or is there some other form of life? If there is an afterlife, what's it like?

The questions are literally endless. And there is no real, concrete answer to any of them, at least not in this life. From my experience, the point of the spiritual struggle that comes out of a life-threatening illness or injury is not to find the answers to these questions; it's to be at peace with the mystery that they represent. That's the acceptance that Dr. Kubler-Ross writes about. The test of faith is to truly accept the lack of an answer—no searching through scriptures for a verse that provides a pat solution or engaging in some ritual or prayer discipline with the thought that an answer can be found there. Remaining faithful and trusting God, while living with and within the mystery, *is* the spiritual aspect of the test brought on by the illness.

Part of this balancing act between your spiritual needs and the patient's is the question of whether or not to involve clergy in facilitating discussions about these issues. It's an easy choice when your loved ones are active members of a faith community. In that circumstance, clergy visits, and most likely visits from members of the temple, mosque, synagogue, or church, are happening naturally and are an important part of your loved ones' support system. But what if you, the caregiver, are the member of a faith community and the patient is not? You, like me, may want to have your pastor visit your loved one. Deciding whether or not to invite a clergy visit on behalf of your loved ones is another one of those delicate balancing acts. You can certainly suggest such a visit to your patients, but if they decline, you should honor that. It gets back to the principle of letting the patient set the agenda.

When MaryKay was initially diagnosed with breast cancer and was to undergo a mastectomy, I asked if she'd be open to having my minister, Rev. Bruce Van Blair, call on her at the hospital. With some reluctance, she agreed, and Bruce was on hand just before they took her to surgery. Afterward, she was very grateful, recalling the depth and tenderness of his prayer. "He was just wonderful," she often commented.

She attended our church a few times during her initial recovery period and again after her recurrence to hear him preach. MaryKay was hospitalized four times between the diagnosis of her recurrence and her death, and each time, without asking her permission, I asked Bruce to visit her because I believed she would benefit from more of his wonderful prayers. She didn't always recall that he'd been there, but when she did, she was grateful for his presence. However, when she was ill at home, she was clear that she would be uncomfortable with a visit from Bruce, and I honored her in that.

I firmly believe in the power of prayer to help restore physical well-being as well as to bring about emotional and spiritual healing. We are living in an era now when a greater understanding is dawning about the link between physical and spiritual well-being. Increasing numbers of scientifically-based studies are considering the role of prayer in medical practice outcomes or the effects of secular meditation in the same setting. Both have shown to have beneficial impacts on the patients who follow either practice, and, based on my experience, I believe that both can help caregivers maintain their own well-being.

Meditation

In the case of meditation, its use has been well-known in modern medicine for decades as a way to reduce stress and stress-related medical conditions. It is also used with increasing frequency by physicians as a "way to prevent, slow or at least control the pain of chronic diseases like heart conditions, AIDS, cancer, and infertility. It is also being used to restore balance in the face of such psychiatric disturbances as depression, hyperactivity, and attention deficit disorder (ADD)."[16] Meditation is also now being regularly used to help patients overcome eating disorders by reconnecting their minds and bodies so they can know when to eat and when to stop.

The practice of meditation has become more streamlined as it is used with greater frequency by an increasing number of caregivers and patients—there's less incense burning and use of mantras in favor of focus on a sound or the mediator's own breath. There are literally dozens of ways to meditate, and that may be a source of confusion for you or your loved one, if you want to try to get the benefits of meditation.

Martha Jensen, a meditation instructor at the University of California, Irvine Medical Center in Orange, California, says it's important for beginners to try out different types of meditation to find the one that's right for them. She says a common mistake that novices make is to try one, not like it, and then dismiss all meditation practices as unhelpful. She recommends that patients try various styles of meditation until they find the one that works well for them, the one they are comfortable with and find easy to practice daily. In addition to finding the right meditation practice, Ms. Jensen says another misconception that beginners need to get past is the idea that meditating will somehow get rid of bad feelings that arise out of difficult experiences. What meditation will do, she says, is open the door to you both learning to cope with the difficult experiences, to become accepting of them.[17]

There are dozens of ways to meditate, many of them now taught through hospitals, medical clinics, and community organizations. If your physician can't make a referral, check with the local hospital or the hospital's social worker, or look in the yellow pages under meditation, mental health services, or wellness. If you can't find someone to teach you and your loved one, here is a sample of a simple meditation method. If you aren't able to complete this practice for twenty minutes, don't worry. Just focus on maintaining a relaxed state for as long as is possible.

- Choose a quiet place.

- Sit upright, as if on a throne, but do not sit stiffly. If the patient cannot sit, any comfortably relaxed position in which breath flows easily will work. Allow your breath to move gently through your body, like a sigh, bringing calmness and relaxation.

- Be aware of what feels closed and constricted in your body, heart, and mind. Let each breath open space within those closed-up places. Let your mind, emotions, and senses expand. Note whatever feelings, images, sensations, and emotions come to you.

- Each time a thought carries you away from your focus (and they will), return to your sense of physical connection to the place where you are sitting and to your breathing. Appreciate your moments of stability and peace. Notice how emotions and thoughts appear and disappear. Focus on your still body and calm breath.

- When you are ready to close your time of meditation, do so gently. Bring your awareness to your location; become aware of the sounds and other sensations around you. Let your mind return to conscious awareness and sit with it for a few moments before moving.

When you have concluded your time of meditation, you don't want to jump up and resume a fast pace of life. Meditation puts you into an altered state of being, and you need to give yourself some moments to come back into the world. It's like having your car idling at a stop sign and then tromping onto the accelerator in order to get up to sixty-five miles per hour as quickly as possible. It's not good for the car, and the same practice in coming out of a meditative state isn't good for you.

Prayer

Dale A. Matthews is a physician who reviewed a variety of scientific studies about the effect of various faith practices on physical well-being and recovery from illness and injury. His study of the results in this field of research contained in *The Faith Factor: Proof of the Healing Power of Prayer* is one of a growing number of books on the subject of how faith affects physical well-being. Here, I want to look at how prayer can be incorporated into your time with your loved one.

Prayer, according to physician Larry Dossey, is not easily defined. In his book *Healing Words: The Power of Prayer and the Practice of Medicine,* Dr. Dossey notes,

> [The word comes from the Latin root word] *precarious*—obtained by begging—and *precari*—to entreat—to ask earnestly, beseech, implore ... but like the 108 names for the Ganges in Hinduism, the classification of prayer can seem endless; theologian Richard J. Foster describes twenty-one separate categories.[18]

Dr. Matthews lists five types of prayer—petitionary, ritualistic, colloquial, meditative, and intercessory. Dr. Dossey's broader list adds also a state of prayerfulness, "an all-pervading sense of holiness and a feeling of empathy, caring, and compassion for the entity in need." Dr. Dossey says that this state of prayerfulness incorporates a deep level of acceptance characterized by the phrase "Thy will be done."[19]

Whether the studies involved people who didn't know they were being prayed for or whether the studies involved the medical team and patients in the prayer, both physicians note that in a significant number of cases—up to 40 percent in one comprehensive study—these studies demonstrated that the subjects had better outcomes or experienced fewer medical problems, such as amount of pain or complications, when prayer was involved. Dr. Dossey's analysis, as well as at least one study cited by Dr. Matthews, point toward more frequently reported benefits when the patients engaged in colloquial prayer (a form of conversation with God) or meditative prayer (contemplation of an idea or concept) or when they were the subject of intercessory prayer from others who prayed for their well-being. Dr. Dossey's state of prayerfulness also tended to demonstrate a greater rate of benefit than for those who engaged in the rote and repetition of ritualistic prayer, who asked for their symptoms to be removed in petitionary prayer, or who did not pray or receive prayers at all.

These studies seem to suggest that prayer that incorporates interaction or personal relationship with God benefits the subjects because they are able to use this kind of prayer to express an acceptance of the divine plan. These types of prayer are different in practice, and apparently in results, from the more institutionalized form of prayer, which has a set of rules about the right way to pray. Still, all of the studies cited by Dr. Dossey and Dr. Matthews merely emphasize what people of faith have known all along—prayer is good for us when we align our physical and intellectual aspects with our spiritual selves.

My spiritual life is my foundation, and prayer is an integral part of my life. I incorporate prayer into all important activities, including caring for a loved one during a major illness. On the other hand, if you're like my sister or my father, this is a problematic issue because it leads you onto uncertain ground. Again, we find ourselves in a delicate situation, in which the needs and beliefs of patients have to be balanced against the needs and beliefs of caregivers.

As a caregiver, I believe the best course is to let your patients lead. If they want to pray with you, then that's what you do, as long as it doesn't violate your personal beliefs. If such an activity poses a problem for you, you will need to let your loved ones know and then find a way in which they can have the resource of prayer in a way that works for both of you. I suspect that patients who are interested in prayer are going to be part of a faith community and will have people there with whom they can pray. If they do not belong to a church, temple, or mosque, you can contact one and probably find someone there who would be delighted to come pray with your loved ones. Hospitals, nursing homes, rehabilitation facilities, and hospice services have chaplains who can be called upon for prayer.

Likewise, intercessory prayer, in which others pray for the healing of someone else, can be a great gift, whether or not you or your loved ones believe prayer is helpful. Dr. Matthews's and Dr. Dossey's books cite numerous examples of the ways in which intercessory prayer benefited patients, regardless of their belief system at the time they were being prayed for or whether they were even aware they were the subject of someone else's prayers. Cyndy, whose story I told earlier, is a dramatic example of how intercessory prayer can benefit patients, even when they don't know they're being prayed for.

Cheryl, my friend who is a college instructor, was surprised when one of her students wanted to pray with her in her classroom after class was over one day. Earlier, Cheryl had told the class that another teacher would be taking over for a few sessions because she was about to undergo reconstructive surgery following her mastectomy.

"I was so surprised," Cheryl recalled. "But I pray, so I thought *why not?*" The young woman took her teacher's hands and prayed for her healing and for God to be present in the surgeon's hands. "It was a beautiful, moving prayer," Cheryl said. "And afterwards, I felt such a deep sense of peace and comfort."

Once you answer the question of whether to incorporate prayer in your time of being with the patient, your next question may well be what to pray. Ritualistic prayers from your faith tradition are always appropriate if they give those praying a sense of comfort in feeling close to God. As Dr. Matthews noted, the three types of prayer that produce the most positive results are contemplative, colloquial, and intercessory. Contemplative prayer, because it involves an individual's focus on a specific concept, such as a word or phrase from sacred text, is best used for times when you or the patient are alone. Intercessory prayer involves someone other than the patient praying. In this form of prayer, the person praying is asking God to be allowed to intercede on behalf of the patient in order to direct God's healing power to the patient. You would offer an intercessory prayer on behalf of your loved one. Colloquial prayer, a conversation with God, is the oldest form of prayer recorded in the Jewish—and therefore Muslim and Christian—tradition, in the conversations between God and Adam in the first book of the Bible.

One other option, if the patient and you are open to it, is to have a time of prayer that can involve a whole circle of close friends and family. The idea is to gather around the patient to pray for healing in whatever way God can bring it into the patient's life. This can be a powerful experience for all concerned, especially when the goal is *not exclusively* to petition for cure. When the prayer circle invites the Spirit's presence into the process for the patient, as well as caregivers, medical team members, and volunteers, an amazing spiritual depth is created that can only benefit the physical aspect of the patient's treatment and care. I have been part of these prayer circles which have involved both the prayers touching the person— a gentle laying of their hands on their loved one—and the prayers and patient being physically distant from each other. Either way, it has been beneficial for all involved, usually in ways that are both anticipated and unexpected.

Samples of Prayers

So, if you're convinced that praying with the patient is a good idea, what words do you use to pray? If you and your loved one are members of a faith community, this is probably not an issue; you'll be familiar with the different types of prayer and comfortable with the process. But if either or both of you aren't familiar with prayer, you may want some general guidelines.

Dr. Barrie Cassileth, a cancer researcher who specializes in studies of alternative and complementary medicines, offers some advice about prayer content in *Cancer Talk* by Selma Schimmel: "The idea that we pray and hope for healing, not necessarily a cure, is important. We need to shift the emphasis. Not 'God, please cure me,' or 'God, why has thou forsaken me?' But rather, 'God, please help me.'"[20]

In praying, as with any conversation, open with a greeting to God.

- "Dear Lord God, we come to you this morning to ask your presence ... " It's up to you whether you pray for a specific outcome—"Please, cure my mother of her Alzheimer's"—or whether you follow the advice of Dr. Cassileth and Dr. Dossey and simply seek that state of prayerfulness—"You know that my mother here is suffering from Alzheimer's. We come to you in prayer to ask acceptance of her condition as you are working out your purpose in her life."

- An example of a general type of prayer seeking the presence of God in the process of dealing with the disease or injury is offered by Dr. Dossey: "May the best possible outcome prevail."[21]

- Another general type of prayer came across the Internet, forwarded by a friend from my church: "Dear God, bless my loved one in whatever it is that you know she may be needing today. May my loved one's life today be full of your peace, presence, and power as she seeks a closer relationship with you."

- I have frequently used a brief prayer that asks God to grant comfort and peace of mind to patients and their loved ones. If you are Christian, I believe it's necessary to offer your prayer in Jesus' name. I also believe that it's also important to thank God for his presence and then to close with an amen, which is a one-word affirmation of the importance of the prayer.

- Twelve-step programs, starting with Alcoholics Anonymous, have traditionally used the serenity prayer, which you might find useful. It's a variation on the peace and comfort prayer: "Dear God, give us strength to accept with serenity the things that cannot be changed. Give us courage to change the things that can and should be changed. And give us wisdom to distinguish one from the other."

- Dr. Lauren Artress, a member of the clergy staff at San Francisco's Grace Cathedral, quotes a Buddhist prayer in her book *Walking a Scared Path: Rediscovering the Labyrinth as a Spiritual Tool.* I've rewritten it slightly to incorporate the example of a caregiver praying with her mother who has Alzheimer's disease. The prayer, which Rev. Artress credits to Stephen Levine, is written in the first person singular—I. "May my mother and I each dwell in the heart. May my mother and I each be free from suffering. May my mother and I each be healed. May my mother and I each be at peace."[22]

- A longer prayer but one that is still of a colloquial nature and invokes the state of prayerfulness might be: "O Great Creating God, we ask you to be close to us as my mother is struggling with her illness and treatment. Let the light of your love and mercy shine in this dark time of fear, anger, and distress. Bless all those who are working to help in my mother's healing, that they may do their work with the great skill you have given them. Hold us gently in your hand, that we may know the peace of mind and comfort of your loving presence. Thank you for being with us as we pray in Jesus' name. Amen."

- The following are a series of prayers for healing that were given to me by a friend from St. Michael and All Angels Episcopal Church in my hometown. Like the prayers already mentioned, these too can be adapted so you are praying for or with someone else, such as "We do not know what this day will bring to my mother ... "

- "I do not know what this day will bring to me, O God, but make me ready for whatever will be. If I am to stand, help me stand bravely. If I am to sit, let me sit quietly. If I am to lie low, help me to do so patiently."

- "God before me, God behind me, God above me, God beneath me. God walking beside me."

- "The body that is giving me pain, O Best of Healers, make whole. The heart that is fearful and hard, make warm beneath your hand."

- "You are the God that heals me. I am your beloved child. You are the God that heals me. I am your beloved child. You are the God that heals me. I am your beloved child."

- "God of tenderness and strength, you have led me to this day. Stay with me as I pray through this time of change, trouble, and pain. Bless this place and those who will care for me today. Bless my home and all whose love sustains me. Fill my heart with tenderness and love."

- "Angels of God, guard me this night and quiet the powers of darkness. Let me rest in the shelter of the Spirit. Then, God of Grace, grant me a safe lodging, a holy rest, and peace at the last."

Whether you are struggling with an issue of how much conversation about spiritual issues you should share with your loved one or whether clergy visits and prayer are appropriate, I want to reemphasize my belief that caregivers need to take their lead from their patients. Remember that your spiritual needs and practices are not the same as your patients' needs, beliefs, and practices. As much as you want them to share your faith, you cannot—and should not—force it on them. Or as much as you don't want them to share *their* spirituality with *you,* then you will need to find a way to make space for them to share their thoughts on these important issues with someone else. As it is their bodies that are ill or injured and therefore their choice as to what medical treatments they will accept or reject, so it is their souls and also their choice as to how they will tend to its well-being.

What You Can Do

It seems a bit odd to list what you can *do* after advising you that your greatest gift—the richest blessing you have to offer—is to *be* with your patients. However, there are lessons to be learned, and here is a recap of them for you to consider.

- *Listen*—Three of the physicians that I quoted in this chapter—M. Scott Peck, Rachel Remens, and Elisabeth Kubler-Ross—had the same piece of advice: listen to your loved ones. It's the greatest gift you can give them. Remember Dr. Siddall's active listening and Rev. Beadle's three-point rule—let them talk; listen; and you can't fix it, just listen. This is your primary job when you are with your loved ones. Let them set the agenda—don't force your issues into their process.

- *Visitors*—Personal visits, phone calls, and notes are all important to keep people who are ill feeling connected to the life they had before the medical crisis. Remember how abandoned Emma felt because her tennis group didn't stay in contact. In *Tuesdays with Morrie*, Morrie Schwartz, who is dying, says, "Here's how my emotions go ... when I have people and friends here, I'm very up. The loving relationships maintain me."[23] Encourage people who are outside the inner circle to stay in contact with your loved one. If they are uncomfortable being physically present, urge them to make phone calls and send a note from time to time.

- *Time Limits*—This comes up in a variety of ways. The first is a good sort of problem to have—managing many people who want to visit your loved ones. The concern should be your patients' physical need for rest versus their need to have visitors. If your loved ones are strong and want company, then it's considerably less of an issue than if they are physically weak. You or your loved ones may also want to establish a priority list when their strength is at a low ebb because there may be days when someone will have to make choices as to who gets to visit and make use of their limited strength. That may get down to deciding whether the relative from out of state or the college classmate from across town spends time with your loved one. It's also a good idea to limit the duration of the visits when energy is low. A visit doesn't have to last an hour or more to be meaningful. Ten minutes of time really focused on the patient is also worthwhile. Another area where time—and your patience—comes up is in allowing patients time to prepare themselves for visitors. It may take them a while to maneuver the walker or crutches so they can answer the door. I inadvertently caught one friend off guard when I showed up at her house unexpectedly. (Shame on me!) Her hair never properly grew back from surgery and chemotherapy to fight her brain tumor, which I was unaware of at the time. She arrived at the door after I'd rung the bell a couple of times, breathless and embarrassed, apologizing that she had to take a moment to put on her wig. I was doubly embarrassed to have put her in such a predicament. A side rule here is to always call before visiting.

- *Your Habits/The Patient's Condition*—You need to look at your personal habits in light of your loved one's medical condition and be willing to change them or set them aside when you are with the patient. Back in the seventies, when smoking had not been banned anywhere, my mother was hospitalized as a result of her colon cancer treatments. One friend came to visit, plopped herself down on my mother's bed—a jarring way to start a visit—and lit a cigarette. It never occurred to the friend to consider how her smoking would affect a woman suffering such extreme reaction to chemotherapy that she'd been hospitalized. Your loved one is functioning in new circumstances, and you need to look at your normal behavior to determine if it's appropriate now or if it needs to be changed. These behaviors include smoking, drinking, when and what you watch on television, how loud or soft to play music or the TV, food choices, and even how you physically interact. The best guide is to ask the patient what will and won't work. If you're desperate to watch the playoff game on the TV and he or she is not up to it, then accept the fact that you'll miss seeing that event while you're with the patient (recording devices for TVs were invented for just such circumstances). Likewise, if your loved one wants to watch the game and you don't care about it, be willing to watch. Instead of resisting the idea, savor the time spent sharing something so enjoyable to him or her.

- *Meals*—I talked quite a bit about meals in the preceding lesson, but since this is such an important way of sharing yourself and your support, there are a few more ideas to consider. If your loved ones have diet restrictions based on their condition, one of the most loving things you can do is to honor those restrictions when you're with them. If the rule is no meat, don't fix yourself a big, juicy steak like they used to enjoy while they are sitting at the same table with a tofu burger. If they're eating tofu, then while you're with them, suspend your need for steak and try tofu. Likewise, there may be restrictions on food handling in order to minimize exposure to infection. These restrictions need to be honored too. It may seem ridiculous to you that you can't slice the meat and the salad greens with the same knife, but their lives may depend on you taking those restrictions seriously. When your patients are dealing with nausea as a side effect, be sensitive about what kinds of food you bring them or prepare for them in their home. If the smell of certain foods is particularly sickening to them, those foods should be banished without a second thought. Don't insist they try your fabulous chicken soup when what they're asking for is yogurt. The chicken soup may make them ill.

- *Rituals*—These are small sacred memorials that can be created throughout your loved one's treatment. Rabbi Kamin writes: "Whatever the ritual, however the devotion, an affinity with God is a kinship with mortality. It distills time—slowing the rush, softening the fear, calming the soul."[24] Dr. Remens describes rituals as "caring made visible."[25] For more than twenty years, she has assisted her patients to gather their inner circle in a ceremony to prepare them for an upcoming treatment—surgery, radiation, or chemotherapy. Another good time for ritual or a ceremony is when patients want to memorialize a specific time—the last radiation treatment, the last physical therapy session, or the first day out of the house or back at work. If a time is worth noting, include your thanks to God, along with an expression of the patients' feelings and some small physical reminder of what is being memorialized. This little ceremony can include the expressions and tokens from the inner circle as well. In Dr. Remens's ceremony, she has each person bring a small object to relate how that object symbolizes a quality they used to overcome a crisis, and then each participant gives it to the patient. I very much wanted our circle of three college friends to do that for Cindy before she underwent a bone marrow procedure in which she was to be given a hugely potent and toxic dose of chemotherapy. My two other friends demurred, fearing they wouldn't know what to say and that they might cry and upset her. Cindy wasn't too enthusiastic about it either. So I took the small polished stone I had hoped to use in the ritual, wrote a note explaining its significance, and left it on her front doorstep in a little gift box where she found it on her way to the hospital. She kept the stone with her throughout her three-week hospital stay. My point is that providing the support of the ceremony is what's important, and, as with so many other aspects of your support of your loved ones, you have to let them decide what they can accept.

- *Reading*—There was a time in our culture—before the advent of electronic entertainment—when we read to one another, a lovely way of sharing our time together. If your loved ones are in a condition in which reading on their own is difficult or impossible, a gift that you can easily provide is reading to them. I read to my grand-mother when she was nearly paralyzed from Parkinson's disease. She enjoyed having access to the books I brought along—Erma Bombeck was her favorite author—and I treasure the memories of the time we spent in that way. Ms. Bombeck wrote hilariously funny books about her life as a homemaker and mother. Reading her books was a way in which I could provide my grandmother with the medicine of laughter. Remember that this is a gift for your patients, so your choice of reading material has to focus on their likes and dislikes, not yours.

- *A Healing Garden*—This can be any place in which your loved one can be outdoors—or see the outdoors—and enjoy the peace and serenity of natural surroundings. This can be a home garden or courtyard, or it may be installed or already exist in an institutional setting such as a hospital or rehabilitation facility. The idea is for your loved ones to enjoy the beauty of the garden, whatever its size, and be able to release some of the stress of their medical condition and treatment. One reason for the stress reduction is that such a garden, designed specifi-cally to be restful and serene, can become a place where they have the opportunity to exercise some control over their choices. In their world, where control of so much of their lives is in the hands of the medical team, having the choice of "whether to sit in sun or shade makes a difference in reducing stress, especially when people are ill," according to Naomi Sachs, a Santa Fe-based archi-tect and proponent of healing gardens.

- *Reminiscing*—Sharing memories with your loved ones is a gift because it can help them to stay in touch with the whole person that they still are. In dealing with their present condition and its focus on their illness or injury, they may begin to lose sight of that *other* person, the individuals they were before this crisis. *Remember when*... can be the key to help them reopen the door to who they are through visits to events from their past. When my sister was very ill, I would gather up photos from around her house and sit by her bedside talking about our memories of people and events. It's a quiet process, and you may well need to allow for some times of silence. Be cautious in engaging in this process that you don't set it up in such a way that merely reminds your patients of what they once were and will never be again. It's another place of balancing recollections of the past to provide a sense of wholeness against reminders of what the patient's life will no longer include.

- *Plans for the Future*—Hope and optimism are important to your loved one's progress, and making future plans is one way to incorporate these qualities into your time with the patient. As always, let the patient give you your cues. At one point, MaryKay and I talked about the two of us renting a house in Tuscany for a week (maybe even two) after she finished with her cancer treatments. After several months, she sadly told me that she didn't think that even when she was done with the chemo and radiation that her stamina would be sufficient to make the long trip. So we spent some time thinking up an alternative and came up with a week (or maybe even two) in a house in the California wine country in the Napa, Sonoma, or Santa Ynez valleys. We looked at magazine articles and considered lots of possibilities, which made that trip planning time together very enjoyable for both of us. This is another one of those balancing acts in which the optimism that inspires the future planning is within reasonable and realistic boundaries. For instance, my sister liked to talk about participating in events dedicated to breast cancer, such as the local running of the Komen Foundation's Race for the Cure, held in September, or the Avon Three-day event from Santa Barbara to Malibu. "I'm going to the Race for the Cure, even if you have to push me around the course in my wheelchair," she'd say. Her goal for the Three-day was to once again attend the closing ceremony in which the participants are welcomed to the finish line like the conquering heroes they are. In neither case did she talk about being a racer or one of the walkers who covers the seventy-five miles. For her, it was enough to look forward to participating in these events on her level.

LESSON NINE:
EMOTIONAL/ PSYCHOLOGICAL SUPPORT

February 5, 1998

MaryKay is very much tuned into doing this next week differently from the last time. That first round of this new, powerful chemo was such a disaster—she was wiped out by the side effects, as much as her inability to take even the most basic steps to offset them. The level of denial/self-sabotage was scary. But now, she's focused on drinking lots of fluids, and, having seen her therapist yesterday, she's beginning to understand that, yes, she is depressed. More—or at least equally—importantly, she is beginning to see how that depression plays out in her behavior.

This is one point where you may encounter a good deal of resistance, either your own or your loved one's. But I firmly believe that emotional—or if you prefer, psychological—support from outside the inner circle is a *necessity*. As much as your loved ones can draw strength and encouragement from your loving support, they are going to need outside help in coping with the nonphysical effects of their condition. The more serious the condition and the longer its duration, the more this kind of support becomes crucial to their total well-being. And the same principle holds true for you, the caregiver. Lorna Reed, the USC/Norris Cancer Center board member and cancer survivor, says "the worst part ... is the unknown, but talking to someone you know and trust—someone who has been through it—can really help ease that fear."[1]

The support I'm recommending serves two purposes. First is the empathy factor, the need for patients to talk about their experiences with others who have also gone through the same process. Caregivers can be supportive and sympathetic, but unless they've been treated for the same condition, they cannot truly know what their loved ones are going through. That's where support groups can be valuable assets to patients. And it's the same for you—your friends can sympathize, but it is better for you if you can talk about your feelings and your experiences with other caregivers who have been in a similar situation.

The second form of outside assistance comes from licensed counselors or psychotherapists. A relationship with a skilled counselor/therapist gives either you or the patient a further safe haven to examine your deepest feelings as you both live through the medical crisis. For the patient, it is frequently true that these feelings are not appropriate to share with family or friends, as the source of the emotions may be tied to those very inner circle relationships. Likewise, the source of your emotional upheaval will be tied to the patient, so it is a good idea for you to have someone other than the patient, or even other caregivers, with whom to discuss your emotions. I believe it is extremely important to have an outsider who is trained in helping sort out the emotional impact of the issues that surround both patient and caregiver. A capable therapist can help you or your loved one get in touch with these deep feelings that you wouldn't feel safe sharing with anyone else. In doing so, the counselor or therapist can facilitate the process of healing through reconciliation of relationships and release of regrets.

There's a medical reason for seeking this kind of support, particularly that which is offered in a support group of people who are in similar circumstances, be they patients or caregivers. Sharing experiences with a support group, whether you are a patient or a caregiver, has been proven to be physically beneficial by reducing stress. People who attend support groups or receive professional counseling have demonstrated higher levels of well-being, less anxiety, and less depression than people in similar circumstances who don't seek such outside help. These beneficial results have been demonstrated several times in a wide variety of studies. A Stanford University Psychiatrist, Dr. David Spiegel, made a long-term (more than twenty years) study of cancer patients and discovered that not only were the patients in support groups better off emotionally, but they reported experiencing less pain than the patients who did not attend support groups.

Initially, Dr. Spiegel's study, which was released in 1977, found that the support group patients lived an average of eighteen months longer, a result that he concluded could not be related to any factor other than attendance at these group meetings.[2] However, subsequent studies made in the nineties did not show the increased longevity that Dr. Spiegel's study showed. One reason for the disparity may be the change in cancer treatments between the seventies and nineties.

The new studies continue to show benefits from attending support groups. There were 235 women diagnosed with metastatic breast cancer in the latest study conducted by Dr. Pamela Goodwin of the University of Toronto. These are women whose cancer had spread beyond the initial breast tumors. The 158 who were assigned to support groups did not show increased longevity beyond the 77 who received only medical treatment. However, Dr. Goodwin notes, like Dr. Spiegel, that they did report less pain and less emotional distress.[3]

Support Groups

Support groups are usually the more easily accessed—and the least costly—of this outside help. These can be groups of up to twenty people (although most groups try to keep membership at six to twelve people) who meet regularly—usually weekly— to talk about their personal experiences and concerns. These kinds of groups are founded on twin principles of honesty and confidentiality in order to create a place in which members can safely share their feelings about their experiences. Fees, if any are charged, are nominal. These groups can be led by a medical or a mental health professional or by a lay person who has lengthy experience in dealing with the medical condition. Group meetings, which last from sixty to ninety minutes, may emphasize emotional support through sharing of experiences, or they may feature a speaker who has a particular expertise that is related to the condition, such as nutrition, legal issues, or new therapies. Group members also support one another by sharing information about resources.

There are a variety of support groups: there are support groups for the patients, there are support groups for family members and friends (the caregivers), and there are support groups for specific family members, such as groups for parents, siblings, or children of patients. These support groups for specific family members may not be as plentiful as the general family groups or the patient groups. Most often, these groups for parents or children can be found in urban and large suburban areas. Support groups are usually sponsored by the hospitals and clinics where the diseases or injuries are treated or local chapters of national organizations that focus on that particular condition. Larger churches also may have these kinds of groups.

I know the idea of walking into a room full of strangers and sharing your very personal feelings—or listening to these strangers talk about theirs—is an intimidating prospect. The only way to overcome your fear is to give it a try. Don't feel that you are required to talk at all during your first visit or two—although you probably will be asked to introduce yourself.

I was surprised the first time I joined a church support group. My plan was to introduce myself and let it go at that. But I wanted them to know that it was because of my sister's illness that I was there. And once I said that, it was as if a small dam gave way, and I shared some of my feelings of grief at the return of her cancer and my fear that she would not be able to overcome it again. No one interrupted. No one prompted me. They just let me say what was on my mind—and heart—and when I stopped talking, I was asked if I had anything else I needed to share. That was enough for that point in time, so the other members of the group took their turns. It was a remarkably easy group of people to talk to and listen to. I still participate with them in their regular meetings.

I encourage you to find a support group because they are just what their names describe—a group of people who can support you with encouragement, information, shared techniques for coping, and assistance when you have difficult choices to make. The easiest way to get involved in a group when you're feeling a bit intimidated is to give yourself permission to just show up and listen and then see what happens after that.

Some patients understand and readily accept the idea that a

support group will help them as they make their medical journey. Some do not. Given my belief in the importance of this kind of outside help, it was, at times, frustrating for me to see my sister initially resistant to this idea. She went through her initial bout with breast cancer not participating in a support group for cancer patients at our local hospital. MaryKay gave it a couple of tries but decided the breast cancer group was a bit of a bore. She said she didn't want to have to listen to stories of women who were still ill while she was recovering. (Remember that she went through this phase believing that her cancer was just a speed bump on the road of life.) In this group, a few women tended to take over the conversation and repeat—endlessly in MaryKay's opinion—their stories of suffering. As much as I could see the benefit of her attending, there was nothing I could say that would alter her point of view.

Her attitude changed when she was emotionally reeling in the aftermath of the diagnosis of recurrence. She became a regular member of a breast cancer support group and said she really missed the support the other women had to offer when she couldn't attend. What she found out the second time around—that perhaps her mind-set on recovery during her initial experience didn't allow for—was that she and the other women spoke a common language, one they could not share with their families or friends. This level of support that MaryKay discovered grew naturally out of the fact that everyone in the group had shared her experiences.

I have met with one interesting caregiver support group that was created in order to get the spouses of the caregivers to attend a patients' support group. The women became acquainted in the hospital's waiting room and got the chaplain to help them set up their group. They then told their husbands that there would be a patients' group meeting at the same time. It was a "Why don't you sit in with that group while I'm at mine?" type of request made to the patients, and it worked! Ironically, the caregiver group has ceased meeting, but the patients' group is going strong and growing.

Psychotherapy

What exactly is this other outside professional help that I'm recommending? It goes by a variety of names—counseling, therapy, or psychotherapy. I am using these terms in a very general way and somewhat interchangeably to describe systematic help that you or your loved one can obtain from a mental health professional.

Psychotherapy can be used to treat individuals, couples, or families who are experiencing emotional or behavioral problems. It is also used, along with medications, to treat individuals with mental illnesses. In most types of psychotherapy, patients discuss their problems with a therapist or counselor one on one, although there are also treatment regimens for couples or families and there is also a group therapy treatment model. The therapist or counselor's role in psychotherapy is to try to gain an understanding of the patient's problem and then to help this person to change the thoughts, feelings, or behaviors that are causing the distress.[4]

When most people think of psychotherapy, they think of the bearded psychiatrist taking notes while the patient lies on a couch conducting a monologue. The use of the couch and the monologue is part of one type of therapy—psychoanalysis. For the most part, the other types of therapy revolve around an interaction between the patient—sometimes also called a client—and the therapist or counselor. Ideally, the atmosphere for these meetings is easy, relaxing, and informal. The sessions are held in an office that's usually set up to resemble a comfortable living room or study. The therapists and patients discuss between them the problems that the patients are dealing with, and the therapists will assist by either suggesting some new ideas for coping or by leading their patients to a new understanding of how they might more successfully cope with their emotional problems.

Individual therapy can fall into one of several categories, depending on the type of professional who is providing the therapy and the type of therapy model that's being used. In the "What You Can Do" section at the end of this lesson, there is a list of the different types of mental health professionals who provide counseling and therapy, along with suggestions for picking a counselor or therapist who will be a good fit for you or your loved one. The following is a general list of the types of psychotherapy available to you and your patient.

- *Psychoanalytic therapy* is also described as "the talking cure" because it is based on having patients talk about whatever is on their mind. These are the therapists who use a couch. The philosophical basis of this approach is that much of human behavior emerges from our unconscious mind, so by talking, patients can reveal what their "unconscious needs, motivations, wishes, and memories [are] in order to gain conscious control of [their lives]."[5]

- *Psychodynamic therapy* looks at important relationships and experiences from childhood to the present. The goal is to resolve emotional and behavioral problems. It can be either long- or short-term.

- *Interpersonal therapy* focuses on the patient's current life and relationships within the family and other environments.

- *Group therapy* is similar to, but also different from, the support groups that I mentioned earlier. A support group is not based on a psychological or mental health treatment regimen. It is voluntary, meaning the participants come as they feel the need. A support group may or may not be run by a therapist or mental health professional. Group therapy is based on a treatment model and is always directed by a mental health professional. This kind of therapy combines people with similar problems into one group under the professional's guidance. A therapy group is somewhat like a support group in that members of the group discuss their individual issues and provide support for one another.

- *Family therapy* involves discussions and problem-solving sessions with members of a family, sometimes in a group setting and sometimes individually.

- *Couple's therapy* focuses on the relationship. The goal is to enhance the relationship by understanding how individual conflicts are expressed in the way in which the couple communicates.

- *Play therapy* is a technique for establishing therapeutic communication with young children.

- *Behavioral therapy* uses an array of learning methods to help an individual change problematic thinking patterns that lead to undesirable behavior patterns. Some of the methods are stress management, biofeedback, and relaxation training. Anger management is a form of behavioral therapy.

- *Other treatments,* which are also known as adjunct treatment, may be used in combination with the therapies listed above. These include occupational, recreational, or creative therapies.

Psychological counseling is not always covered by health insurance, which is a key issue because it's expensive on a private basis. However, there are numerous sources for therapy where the cost is based on the patient's ability to pay. Check for referrals with the hospital or clinic where your loved one is being treated. Many communities—again most typically the urban and large suburban areas—have non-profit organizations that provide low-cost counseling. Organizations such as the YMCA and Family Services may offer sliding-scale fee services. Large churches, again, can also be a good source for finding such services, although the counseling offered would obviously have a spiritual component because it is church-based. Veteran's Administration hospitals and clinics are another place to look for affordable counseling. Teaching hospitals, where physicians are trained, are also settings in which you are likely to find affordable individual or group therapy.

In addition to joining a support group, MaryKay's oncologist had also recommended that she talk to a therapist, a woman who was also a breast cancer survivor. Again, during her initial diagnosis and treatment, MaryKay was even less interested in visiting the therapist than she was in the breast cancer support group. But as she did eventually recognize the importance of the support group during her recurrence. When she allowed herself to meet with the recommended therapist, she again found someone who spoke her language because of their common experience with breast cancer. More importantly, she also found someone with whom she could talk about the concerns that she didn't want to share with her family, closest friends, or even the support group.

Caregivers Need Outside Support Too

I want to reiterate my opening thought that this type of outside help is good not just for the patient but for the caregivers as well. While you're supporting your loved one, you need to be able to share your feelings with others or with a therapist who can help *you* sort out *your* feelings.

During my sister's illness, I used both the church-based support group and a therapist, which was the polar opposite of my experience when my mother was ill twenty-five years earlier. When Mom was sick, the idea that I might need support never occurred to me. At that time, I was in my late twenties, and my mind-set was that *she* was the patient and my job was to support *her*. It seemed selfish for me to think in terms of support that I might need. So I sought none, even though I was suffering from intense migraine headaches. It never occurred to me that my need to talk out my feelings was in any way related to the crippling headaches.

In those days—the early seventies—support groups weren't necessarily readily available, and professional counseling was outside my frame of reference. I had a job, a husband, two small children, and a sick mother, and that occupied all of my time. It wasn't until the day of Mom's funeral that a window opened up to the possibility that I might have asked for support for myself. My closest high school friend came to the funeral, and in the informal receiving line that developed afterwards at the church, she grabbed me by both my hands with an appalled expression on her face. "Oh, Joannie," she said. "I feel so awful. I didn't know your mom was sick. *Why didn't you call me so I could help you?*" It was then that I realized how isolated I'd been in dealing with my mother's illness and death.

That memory has stayed with me over the years, and I

have learned that selfishness and selflessness are complex ideas that can seem to be in conflict at times. It is *not* selfish to take care of yourself so that you can help someone else. Selflessness, in which you pour yourself out endlessly for someone else until you have nothing left to give him or her, in the end doesn't help either of you, if you are exhausted or become ill yourself in the process. It is as important for you as for the loved one whom you are supporting that you find support for yourself. Understanding this principle, I have become increasingly conscientious about seeking emotional or psychological support for myself as I care for a loved one who is seriously ill.

At the time of my sister's recurrence, I had just started working with Margaret, a talented and sensitive therapist. Initially I began seeing her for assistance with issues related to my desire to retire from the family business, in which my sister, father, and brother-in-law were all still active. But once MaryKay's condition became apparent, my focus with Margaret shifted from retirement issues—since that was precluded by the necessity for me to support my sister by staying involved in the business—and on to the lessons I needed to learn in order to be fully present to her. It was through Margaret's guidance that I learned about *being* with MaryKay, about patience, and about my feelings about the wider issues of mortality.

At the same time I was working with Margaret, I was blessed with a close circle of female friends at my church. We started out as a randomly assembled group that was to share our thoughts and experiences during a women's retreat held just a month after MaryKay was diagnosed with her recurrence. Of course, MaryKay's condition was in the forefront of my sharing, but the other women had their own equally deep and pressing issues as well. Our experience on that weekend was so wonderfully supportive for all of us that we have remained together as a group, gathering monthly to continue sharing our thoughts and feelings as our lives progress.

I relied on this group for my support rather than the hospital-based support group for families not because I disliked the hospital group but because this smaller group functions within the same spiritual realm that I do, and that's very important to me. As a patient needs a support group of other patients who all speak the same language, so I chose to find my support with this group of eight women who speak my spiritual language.

Denial

If you—the patient and caregiver—are not people who regularly work with a counselor, the idea of emotional/psychological support is going to be foreign and will probably be resisted initially. Our culture still puts a negative cast on working with therapists—however skilled and well-trained they may be—to help deal with feelings. It's perceived as being silly or unimportant because such things cannot be physically seen. In this line of thinking, an invisible, emotional wound can't be as serious—and therefore in need of as much attention—as a visible, physical wound. As a result, some people find it impossible to assign the same importance to scars that can't be seen as they do the outward appearance of a traumatic injury.

Further, there's a sense that people who need this kind of help are crazy or weak, unable to pull themselves up by their bootstraps in the best American tradition. The recent Robert De Niro/Billy Crystal movies, *Analyze This!* and *Analyze That!,* and the hugely popular television show *The Sopranos* all use the reluctance of tough guys—the central figures are both Mafia Dons—to seek psychological help as their comedic themes. While Hollywood's wry and sly look at this issue is amusing, the resistance factor is very real because there is fear on the part of the individuals who need this kind of outside support. The fear is simply that once they start examining their feelings, they will open a whole Pandora's box of inner monsters that were better left locked up.

Any of these negative attitudes can facilitate the kind of denial my sister experienced during her initial treatment cycle, in which she convinced herself that she didn't need a support group or a therapist. That denial was shared also by her husband, Chuck, and their son, even after her recurrence when she did seek outside help. Both ultimately spent some time with a therapist, but neither decided to use the services of the local family support group or the group for teenagers whose parents have cancer.

In my nephew's case, I believe that part of the difficulty was in the very fact that he was a young teenager at the time of her illness. Teens have two goals in life after the drive for food, shelter, and sex: to *not* be like their parents (or any other adults) and to *not* stand out in their peer group. He was already standing out in ways he couldn't control because his mother had cancer. Given this mind-set, it's logical that his desire to further distinguish himself by being part of a support group or meeting regularly with a therapist was going to be very limited.

I think my nephew and lots of other teenagers simply can't envision themselves in that circumstance. ("Sorry. Can't hang out. Gotta go see my therapist.") It's a pity because I think that if they can overcome the antipathy, they would find the ability to talk about their feelings with support groups or counselors to be very helpful in coping with a sick parent or sibling at home. A support group provides an opportunity for them to be with others who are like them, a peer group of kids who share the experience of an ill loved one.

The avoidance of support groups or therapy can leave your patients without an appropriate place to express their feelings of fear and anger. A young woman who is a member of my church choir found herself without an outlet for her feelings as she was being treated for breast cancer. Her behavior over the few years of her membership in the church had been problematic for other members because she was the kind of person who had a poorly-developed sense of boundaries. Her occasionally inappropriate behavior tended to make people avoid her, including the other breast cancer survivors in the congregation. While they might have been able to offer the support she needed, they did not want to find themselves in a close personal discussion with her. Their decision was understandable, but it also left this woman isolated.

Needing to express her anxiety, she chose to do so one morning in choir rehearsal. The silence was deafening after she stood up to tell the assembled choir members about her surgery and difficult recovery process and her fear of the upcoming radiation treatments and reconstruction of her breast. I felt so sorry for her that she was experiencing such trials seemingly without support, but at the same time, I was appalled that she'd chosen this group of twenty men and women—none of whom were particularly close to her—with whom to share these deep feelings. Fortunately, our music minister realized her level of desperation and got the senior pastor involved. He in turn steered her to the breast cancer support group at the local hospital.

The rule of thumb in dealing with resistance or denial is the same as for other issues. You can see the problem and recommend the resource once, but if your patients choose not to act on your advice, you cannot force them to do what *you* think is going to be good for *them*. As I've said before, this is their process. As it is their process, you must leave it to them to decide how they will handle it. Your job is to take care of yourself so you can give the best of what you have to offer in supporting the patient. Seek out and use the outside help you need, and let your patients do what they think is appropriate for them.

Finding a Therapist, Counselor, or Support Group

If you live in an urban area or a suburb, finding a therapist or counselor is simply a matter of pulling out the yellow page phone directory and looking under *counseling services, therapists,* or *support groups.*

The patient's medical team members, especially the lead physician, will be a likely source of suggestions for both therapists and support groups, as will the hospital or clinic at which the patient is being treated. If your loved one suffers from a condition for which there is a national organization, such as the Lung Association, the Heart Association, and so on, your local chapter may also provide a referral to support groups in your area.

Another place to find lists of therapists or counselors could be through your health insurance carrier's list of accepted providers. If you are in a health maintenance organization (HMO), there is also a list of providers available there, if the therapists are not already in place in the HMO's local clinic.

The local chapter of the American Medical Association, the American Psychiatry Association, or the American Psychological Association can all provide you with lists of practitioners in your area. And don't forget to check with the VA if you or your loved one is a veteran of military service.

There is a similarity between the way in which you would find a therapist and the process of finding a support group because in both cases it needs to be a comfortable fit for you in order to be beneficial. You're looking for help and support, and if you can't work well with the person or people who are providing it, you're not going to find the help you need. Be choosy. Support groups are like individual therapists in that they have distinct personalities. Be willing to give a group a try for a few sessions—two to four—but if you're not getting the support you need, you also need to be willing to find a group where you can get it.

What You Can Do

The activity suggested here is about finding the support that's going to work best for you. For that reason, it's a good idea to know what questions to ask potential counselors/therapists:

- *Credentials*—What is their education? Did they attend a school accredited by an organization such as the American Psychological Association? Are they licensed in your state? Do they belong to a professional organization that accredits based on professional expertise, such as the American Psychiatry Association, the American Psychotherapy Association, or the International Psychoanalytic Association?

- *Experience*—How much experience have they had in working with people with needs similar to yours or the patient's? For instance, MaryKay's therapist specialized in cancer patients and was herself treated for breast cancer. While having someone that specialized can be a great help to the patient, it's not absolutely necessary. A counselor with a background of working with patients who are facing a variety of health crises will be equally helpful because so many of the therapeutic dynamics are the same.

- *Intensity and Duration*—What kind of a treatment model do they use? How often do they envision meeting with you, and over what period of time? Some therapists use treatment models that are quite intense and might require you to meet with them a couple of times of week. As the prospective patient, you need to decide what will and won't work for you in getting the help the therapist has to offer. The same holds true for the duration of the therapy. Many of the sliding-scale fee programs are based on a short-term but intense program that foresees the therapy continuing for no more than eight weeks. On the other hand, some therapists use a plan that envisions a therapeutic relationship that may last for years. What is your idea? Be sure that what you envision for therapeutic support fits with the therapist's treatment model.

- *Cost*—There is a significant difference in cost based on the qualifications, training, and licensing of therapists. Most state licensing requirements are that therapists should at least have earned master's degrees in a related field of study, such as counseling, psychology, or social work. A rule of thumb is that the more training they've been required to undergo, the more their time will cost. This *does not* mean the quality of the therapy should be regarded as being less worthwhile if the individual has had less schooling. There are many, many excellent counselors who hold just the one graduate degree. Likewise, the converse is true; having graduated from medical school does not necessarily confer skill in psychological therapy. Education levels and fees do not always correlate to the level of *counseling skill* that the person possesses.

- *Training*—When you or your loved ones are looking for therapists, you need an understanding of the training that the person has undergone and the license that they've earned:

  1. *Mental Health Counselor.* These therapists go by a variety of names, depending upon how your home state licenses them. They have earned at least a master's degree, had supervised experience, and passed a state exam before being licensed for private practice. If they are certified by the National Board for Certified Counselors, they have passed a standardized national exam. Some designations under which these therapists practice, depending on the state, are Marriage and Family Counselor (MFC) or Marriage, Family, and Child Counselor (MFCC), Licensed Professional Counselor (LPC), or Licensed Mental Health Counselor (LMHC).

  2. *Social Workers.* Sometimes referred to as psychiatric or clinical social workers, they have advanced degrees in social work, have completed a supervised program of field training, and have passed a state test to become licensed. In addition to therapy, social workers are trained in client-centered advocacy, including information and referral to community resources. Some designations under which these therapists practice, depending on the state, are Masters of Social Work (MSW) or Licensed Clinical Social Worker (LCSW).

  3. *Psychoanalysts or psychotherapists.* These therapists must hold a least a master's degree in counseling, social work, or psychology in order to be licensed.

They may or may not hold an additional certification from a professional association, such as the American Psychotherapy Association or the International Psychoanalytic Association.

4. *Psychologists.* These therapists are also called clinical psychologists. In most states, they have completed a doctoral degree from an accredited university with programs in specialized training. A PhD in psychology also requires a period of supervised training working with patients. State licensing requirements generally include passing of a standardized test.

5. *Psychiatric Nurse.* These professionals generally work in therapy programs related to treatment of mental illness.

6. *Psychiatrist.* This person is a medical doctor (MD) who has taken further training in the diagnosis, treatment, and prevention of mental illness. There is a significant difference between the physiological aspects of mental illness, which psychiatrists are trained to treat medically, and the psychological aspects of emotional problems, which are handled through psychoanalysis or psychotherapy. Not all psychiatrists are therapists. Those who offer therapy may do so in conjunction with treating mentally ill patients. Some psychiatrists who are therapists prefer the work of psychological therapy to the pill-pushing side of psychiatry, which treats the physical aspects of mental illness.

7. *Clergy.* Priests, ministers, and rabbis usually take courses in counseling and psychology as part of their religious training so they can offer their congrega-

tion members counseling. Because their licensing focuses on their religious duties, the quality of the counseling may vary substantially, depending on the individual's personality and the quality of the training that he or she has received.

Other Sources of Support

There may be many reasons why you can't find a support group or a therapist to work with. There are other sources, but, in my opinion, none of these will be as effective as a support group or therapist:

- *Books*—Stroll down—or if you're online, scroll down— the aisle of self-help books at your local bookstore and you will find a dizzying array of titles to choose from. Ask your librarian or friends for recommendations, or check online reader reviews for help in selecting a book that can provide help in dealing with your deep feelings. It's difficult, however, even with the best book you can find, to get the interactive responses that a group or a therapist can offer.

- *Online*—The benefit to using an online chat room is that you have the benefit of interacting with people who are in similar circumstances. Online chat rooms dedicated to people who share your same medical condition or circumstances can be very beneficial. But like any other support group, a chat room will have its own personality, so just be sure there's a match there for you. Be wary of general chat rooms, which are not tied to a site sponsored by a recognized institution or organization. The one detriment to any chat room is that because you can't see the others with whom you're chatting, you have no way to truly assess them and the validity of the support they're offering you.

- *Friends*—This is certainly an interactive resource, and one in which you can feel safe because you know who the people are, so it has much to recommend it. It is a great gift to have friends who are willing to support you however they can. One group of my friends took me on an outing to some beautiful flower fields, acres of blooming ranunculas in a nearby town, followed by lunch at a Thai restaurant. We didn't talk about my sister, and so the support was in the form of a wonderful half-day's respite from those concerns. Your friends may be able to offer you similar respite, or they may have had similar life experiences and can support you by sharing what they learned from those experiences, as do the members of my church support group. Their generosity of spirit in offering support on whatever level—and in whatever way—that they can, will definitely be a blessing to you.

LESSON TEN:
SELF-CARE FOR CAREGIVERS

August 11, 1999

What would make me feel better? It's a question that I've lived with for a long time, some sixteen months between MaryKay's diagnosis of recurrence and her death. Taking my emotional pulse and then finding a short-term cure for what ails me is a behavior pattern I have learned, much like a patient of heart disease learns to take their pulse and medicate themselves with aspirin or nitro glycerin. Processing through the denial, anger, fear, and all of the strong feelings that surrounded my grief for her illness and then death, I seemed to be constantly trying to find ways to determine what activity would get me back to a better place, a place closer to equilibrium. Shopping, a good book, a walk, a drive, a glass of wine—a few glasses of wine—garden work, prayer time. There isn't much that I haven't used to medicate my breaking heart.

The diagnosis of a life-threatening disease or event of a serious injury affects not only the patients but also those who love them. Regardless of the prognosis for cure or recovery, the family and friends who are caring for the ill or injured person have great mountains of emotions to climb as they deal with the impact of their loved one's condition. Major illness or injury unpredictably alters the bedrock of the lives of the patients and their families. It may require changes in lifestyle, sometimes permanently, for the caregiver as well as for the patient. It can force the suspension or even the end of a promising career or lead to a move to a new home or even to a care facility. If the caregiver is financially dependent on the patient whose life and future are in jeopardy, the changes can feel like a complete destruction of a lifetime of plans and dreams. The medical crisis is like an earthquake rumbling through the old, taken-for-granted serenity of the normal life expectations of patient and caregiver alike.

In addition to the emotional content, there's also a physical side to this process. Caring for an ill or injured person is much more demanding than it has ever been in the past. Due to changes in our country's health care system, hospital stays are shorter, which means patients are released to their homes requiring a more intense and more technical level of care than ever before.

The short hospital stays also result in home care of much longer duration. The impact of caregiving is more demanding on the caregiver than it has ever been. Spending a month, or even two, attending to ill or injured loved ones who are in the process of recovering their health is a far different experience than providing a higher level of care for a year or for an indefinite period of time.

Short- or long-term, it is all tremendously demanding for

the caregiver. Even in short-duration caregiving, there will be times when it feels like you're being asked to leap across a chasm. At these times, you'll wonder if it's possible to get across safely and to land in one piece on the other side.

This lesson is intended to provide a safety net for you caregivers—the dedicated spouses, life partners, children, brothers and sisters, parents, friends, and neighbors who form the essential support and care team for the patient. The problem is that your needs are often neglected while you focus on the patient. Dr. Elisabeth Kubler-Ross, in her book *Life Lessons*, quoted a woman who had cared for her husband while he recovered from a lengthy illness:

> I realized I felt so selfish to have my own feelings, my own fears. I never thought to say, "Hey, what about me!" That would have felt wrong. I wasn't the patient, who was I to need help? So I kept my mouth shut until I finally cracked.[1]

As a caregiver, you will find yourself at times struggling with the feelings cited by this woman—unexpressed needs, wanting someone to help *you*—while you also very much want to be fully present to and for your loved one whose need is painfully obvious. My personal experience has been that we who are not ill put ourselves under great physical, emotional, and spiritual stress while we're caring for someone else. We simply stop caring about ourselves and risk falling into a pit of our own, once our inner resources have been depleted in the trying process of giving loving support and physical care to the one who is seriously ill or injured.

Tom, a longtime friend, was the sole caregiver for his wife, Beverly, during the last year of her life. Beverly could see that Tom was having trouble coping with the weight of the daily responsibilities for her care, but she wasn't able to convince him that he needed to engage in some active self-care on his own behalf. As one small concession to her concerns, he would take a walk or go to a nearby gym to work out while she was sleeping in the early morning. But once she was not able to sleep for long at regular intervals, he dropped the practice. He confessed later that it wasn't until after her death, when his own health deteriorated, that he was finally able to see what had worried Beverly.

"If I were to be able to go back and change anything about that year," he told me, "it would be that I'd do a better job of taking care of myself. Just being available to her twenty-four hours a day isn't as important as really being able to give all of myself. I probably would have done a better job of that if I'd given myself some time off."

Understanding the Impact

It's not always easy to see how our desire to care for our loved one impacts us in a physical way. It is likewise not easy to make changes to accommodate the extra demands of the care-giving assignment we've taken on. It took my sister's illness for me to be able to see a pattern that I'd developed over the years, which was to get a cold while I was providing care for my mother, grandmother, or mother-in-law. I would dedicate myself to providing the support my loved one needed, but in my subconscious, I must have known the wisdom of giving myself a break for my own self-care. When I didn't consciously provide that break, my body obliged by allowing me to get a cold. At that point, I couldn't be around my ill loved ones—they didn't need to have their medical condition further complicated by my cold germs—and I was just sick enough to have to take a time-out for a couple of days while I recovered. Fortunately, because I finally caught on to the pattern, it was a relatively simple task to make sure I had some time to take care of myself so I didn't have to get a cold.

In Lesson Seven, I mentioned MaryKay's insistence that her husband, Chuck, get out with his friends on the golf course for a weekly game on Saturday mornings. She clearly understood about the need for her most important caregiver to have some time for himself.

One of the dangers that we caregivers face is overloading ourselves. We have jobs, commitments, our homes and families, and now, in the face of a medical crisis, we add caring for our loved ones to our to-do list. Oftentimes, in taking on this new assignment, we fail to take into account the real nature of the new demand and how much of our time and energy it will consume. Barbara Robinson, a resident of Orange County, California, brought her ailing mother to live with their family after her father died. It has proven to be a difficult choice for her: "In all honesty, my mother used to be my best friend, and now there is some resentment."[2]

One of the ways in which you can care for yourself as a caregiver is to *not* try to maintain your pre-crisis schedule along with your new duties as a caregiver. Look at your list of ongoing responsibilities and find some that you can drop for now. Your primary focus will be the patient, and it usually isn't possible to take an unlimited amount of time from work. What else is on the list that you can release on a temporary basis? Are you active in a religious, community, or work-related organization? Once you are thrust into the role of caregiver, it's time to take a leave from those other duties. Let someone else do your volunteer work while you have this more pressing assignment.

My stepmother, Claudette, dropped a number of community and social activities when Dad was diagnosed with non-Hodgkin's lymphoma. She wanted to be able to give him the support he needed, and she determined that her good works in the community and her active social life would both still be available when he was finished with his treatment. She also knew that they both would need all their energy for dealing with the cancer treatments, so she didn't want to expend this precious resource on social activities. "We can always go to dinner parties later," was her observation.

Stress

The most obvious component that comes with the assignment of caregiver is stress. Stress is emotional upset—an inside occurrence—that is the result of pressure from outside. If you think about it, the first four of the five emotional stages described by Dr. Kubler-Ross are responses to stress. In small doses, stress can be beneficial, helping us to overcome a reluctance to do things we need to do. You put off writing that term paper or getting that report done at work, and the stress of the impending deadline—and fear of how the teacher or boss will punish your non-performance—will motivate you into action.

The problem is that our schedules are so overloaded that our lives have multiple stressors, which have a real and measurable impact on our bodies. There is a change in our blood chemistry when we are upset, and that chemical change manifests itself in physical problems. These problems can include headaches (even migraines), stomach problems (even ulcers), muscle pain, joint pain (even arthritis), sleeplessness, depression, inappropriately angry responses, and short-term memory loss. This list includes more serious problems up to heart attack and stroke, if the stress remains consistently high over a prolonged period of time. Burnout is one way in which stress-induced breakdowns by caregivers are described.

Levels of stress are dependent not only on how much there is—how many deadlines and to-do assignments we're dealing with at one time—but also on our ability to affect the source of the stress by our actions. The less control we have, the greater the stress burden feels. The stress of the pending term paper deadline feels far different from the stress of your loved one's illness because you can write the term paper and get rid of that stress but you can't cure your loved one.

More than that, you may be facing a change forced by the medical condition, another element that's out of your control, which makes it a great source of stress. Change, even when you invite it and plan for it, is always stressful because of that element of "little deaths" that comes with it. Change that's forced upon you and the patient by the medical crisis is significantly more stress-filled. Just the fact of an illness or injury means at least a short-term change in the life pattern of the patients and their caregivers—trips to the hospital or treatment facility, sometimes daily; learning to use medical equipment and accommodating it in the home; and new daily regimens of drugs, therapy, and changes of eating patterns. If the condition is chronic or permanently disabling, the change is going to be deeper, and so is the stress that it will cause.

As a caregiver, your stress levels are related to both quantity of assignments—from trying to add the giving of care to your loved ones to what was probably an already full life—and to lack of control. You find yourself suddenly faced with unanticipated and unwelcome lifestyle changes. Perhaps even more stressful is the fact that because you aren't the patient, the ultimate decisions and reactions to treatment are out of your hands. You can advise, support, love, and care for your patients, but *they* are the ones who are making the choices, expressing the anger, experiencing the side effects, and ultimately they will or will not get better. Other than caring for them, you cannot control the outcome of their medical process, and that is extremely stressful until you can reach the point of genuine acceptance of this fact.

Halina Irving, a psychotherapist who specializes in treating patients with chronic and life-threatening illnesses, says one of the key ideas for caregivers to learn is that "they don't have to fix everything. In fact, they *can't* fix everything ... We want so much to fix it, we want to be the bearers of good news, we want to have some control. It's difficult to acknowledge that we cannot cure the disease."[3]

Even when you can get to the point of acceptance of the fact that you can't fix it, you may still experience stress related to the physical demands of being a caregiver and of having *to do* a number of things for your loved one while continuing to maintain your own life. It's a big burden, and the results most likely will be some physical manifestation, such as headaches, neck and back pains, stomach upset, sleeplessness, or more serious physical problems, such as heart problems or a depressed immune system, which leaves you open to illness. Chronic stress has been shown to impair long-term memory, although studies suggest that relief of the stress allows for the affected area of the brain to recover its pre-stress level of recall. This list of physical impacts indicates the significance of the stress that you're experiencing; that you need to pay attention to its presence, its effect on your body, mind, and spirit, and that you also need to take steps to alleviate as much of it as you can.

Managing Stress

The good news is that the physical response to stress, your body's expression of your feelings, can be controlled to the degree that you are able to manage your reaction and response to stress. You can't change the outcome of your loved one's medical treatment, but you can change the way you let that outcome affect you. Accept the fact that this medical crisis has caused you to have some strong feelings—fear, anger, resentment, or frustration, and probably also guilt for having those feelings at all. Selma Schimmel writes, "It's okay. [Serious illness] is an unwelcome intruder in *everybody's* life."[4]

Once you can accept those strong emotions, what do you do with them? You can keep the anger and pain of watching your loved one suffer through debilitating disease or painful treatments on the inside, where it will find some way to express itself in your body, in symptoms listed earlier in this chapter. Or you can find a way to express those feelings, to let them out in a constructive way—such as journaling or joining a support group—so the feelings lose their negative charge, the actual power to cause your body discomfort or even lasting harm.

Another response to mitigate the effect of stress is to shift your attitude toward the circumstances causing it. It's the old adage about deciding whether to think of the glass as being half-empty or half-full. In the face of a life-threatening illness or injury, it certainly is possible to list all the reasons for hopelessness and let the weight of your helplessness in the face of your loved one's condition push you down into the darkness. Or you can shift your perspective and look for the presence of light, wherever it may be occurring. Hope is a powerful motivator and stress-reliever. Recall Dr. Bernie S. Siegel's adopted motto: "In the face of uncertainty, there is nothing wrong with hope."[5]

Along with hope, there are some positive actions you can take to help manage the stress you'll encounter. Some of these ideas are simply listed here to get you thinking about what you can do to lessen your stress. I provide more details about them at the end of this lesson in the section entitled "What You Can Do."

- Get the training you need in order to handle medical equipment or procedures at home.

- Consider outside help to supplement the care you will be giving at home.

- Take regular breaks from your caregiving duties.

- Cultivate—and use—your own support team.

- Be realistic about what you can accomplish.

- Get professional help in dealing with the emotional/ psychological impact of being a caregiver.

- If you have a job outside the home, find ways to lessen your stress at work.

- Make time for play; give yourself opportunities to laugh.

Learning Self-care

Taking care of myself was a process that I had to learn after my sister was diagnosed with cancer. My body kept trying to teach me with the colds that I'd gotten during the illnesses of other loved ones, but it wasn't until her illness that I developed a plan for caring for myself *so that I could care for her.* I called it the dental floss principle because flossing my teeth was one way I could gauge whether or not I was engaging in self-care.

If I was following a good routine that included prayer time, a long morning walk, and a healthy breakfast, I inevitably took the time to floss my teeth every morning. Using the dental floss was an expression of the care of my body, mind, and spirit that I needed to maintain in order to handle the stress of MaryKay's medical circumstance. Included in that caregiving stress was the resulting pressure on my work life, which in turn affected my home life. On the days when I didn't get around to flossing, I noticed I was foregoing other healthy habits as well because I was rushing to do something. Of course, there were the occasional days when an early-morning meeting meant no walk—and usually no floss—but that was okay. It was when the once-every-few-weeks absence of dental floss started turning into an every-other-day event that I'd force myself to slow down and reprioritize so I could get back to the healthier routine.

Another way to look at this principle is to think of yourself as a garden that needs constant attention in order to present your beauty to the garden's visitors. Your many aspects—trees, grass, flowers, shrubs, fountains, and ponds—all need watering, weeding, pest control, and feeding, along with the sun and good soil so you can be at your best. If you neglect your garden, the beautiful plants will die out, and the visitors will only see a barren patch overrun with snails and ugly weeds.

Laura Claverie of New Orleans wrote of her unusual but productive stress relief method in the March 2002 edition of *Food and Wine Magazine:*

> In times of stress, I take comfort in making my favorite Creole or Cajun foods: gumbo, jambalaya, etouffée, and duck ragout. All require a great deal of chopping, my greatest source of tension release...I chop until my hands ache. I sauté until the fragrance wafts across the whole neighborhood and my cast-iron pot is brimming. I am at peace.[6]

For Ellen Rose, owner of the Los Angeles bookstore *Cook's Library,* baking cakes proved to be a sort of therapy for dealing with a more than yearlong rough patch in her life. She said she'd bake one a day, unless it was a really bad day; then she'd bake two. The cakes were then given to a friend or someone whom she thought needed cheering. She credits the cake baking and the relationships those cakes nourished with helping her to deal with the stress. She was performing a concrete task that enabled her ultimately to reach past her despair and loneliness and reconnect with the people who were important in her life—family, friends, and customers.

"I found that in my own life, during my darkest, worst days, my therapy was to bake ... I've always found that [crises are] a great opportunity to learn something new—there's great growth in that," Ms. Rose said.[7]

I understand how this lesson represents a significant shift in focus from the patient to you, the caregiver. But just as you can well understand your importance to your loved ones because of the care *you* give *them,* likewise you need to appreciate your importance to yourself in the care *you* give *you.* Don't discount the necessity of self-care by deciding that you're not worth it, that you can't take time to care for yourself, or that the suggestions for care that I offer here are silly or extravagant. These suggestions come from personal experiences and are consistently cited in the advice given by the experts I've quoted throughout this book. Ms. Schimmel notes of you caregivers that you "deserve more attention than [you] have been receiving, because [your] efforts are vital to the patients."[8]

Giving Yourself a Break

Marcia Schnedler, writing for Universal Press Syndicate, even advocates running away from home for a short time as a means of self-care. She explains that she went from caring for her father in his difficult final months to discovering almost immediately after her father's funeral that her non-smoking husband had lung cancer. "So we ran away from home on a three-night vacation between his pre-operative tests and surgery." The results were so beneficial in preparing her husband for surgery and treatment and her for resuming the role of caregiver that Ms. Schnedler advocates brief, close-to-home getaways as a form of self-care for caregivers.

"These respites can be vital, because more than half of caregivers are under daily stress as they assist loved ones with dressing, moving, eating, and hygiene," she wrote. Ms. Schnedler quoted a study from the National Family Caregivers Association (NFCA), which noted that 46 percent of family caregivers (as opposed to paid professionals) manage medications, change dressings, monitor vital signs, or perform some other type of nursing. The NFCA study found that the majority of people who put in twenty-one hours or more a week as caregivers suffer some form of sleep deprivation, depression, or both. "Another study found that elderly caregivers who are stressed out—particularly those who have [their own] physical problems—have a 63 percent higher mortality rate than their [non-caregiving] peers."[9]

Ms. Schnedler's get-away recommendation is for the caregiver, though she and her husband went together before he underwent surgery:

- Take a twenty-four- to seventy-two-hour trip to someplace close to home.

- Make it an easy, slow-paced trip that is for relaxation, not necessarily sightseeing or other programmed activity.

- Assuage any guilt by checking in regularly by phone with your loved one and the substitute caregiver.

- Try to keep any emotional blackmail in check in the event that the patient is demanding or manipulating for your return. Don't give up on your get-away because the patient is asking for you, doesn't like the way the substitute is caring for him or her, won't eat/ take medication, etc. This is your break to preserve your health and well-being so that when you return home you will be better able to care for your loved one.

My stepmom, Claudette, was fully prepared to care for Dad by herself in his final days. She didn't want anyone else in the house for prolonged periods of time, especially not a stranger. But when Dad fell and she couldn't get him back into bed, she was forced to call the paramedics for assistance, which they graciously and gently provided. At that point, she agreed to have a professional caregiver in for the nighttime hours so she could get some sleep. She understood that if she were to become ill from lack of sleep or injure herself in trying to help him, then control of his care would have to be taken out of her hands. And that was something she absolutely did not want to happen.

The principle of self-care during this time of medical crisis is *so* important. This is one of the most important lessons that I offer to you: *take care of yourself so you can care for your loved one.* Dr. Kubler-Ross, in *Life Lessons,* seconds that idea, urging caregivers to practice the same level of care and compassion on themselves that they offer to the patient for whom they are caring.[10] You *are* worth the time, and you *must* take time for self-care because whatever care you lavish on yourself will allow you to have that much more of yourself to give to your loved one.

One note of caution, based on personal experience, don't be hard on yourself about letting self-care slip from time to time. I used the dental floss principle to gauge when I was slipping in my responsibilities to myself and then made the necessary changes. You will probably not be able to consistently maintain a good regimen of healthy behaviors given the demands you are responding to. When you do get off track from your plan for yourself, note it and make the changes you need to get back on track. Don't engage in recriminations and beat yourself up for having slipped. It's a natural human behavior; every so often, we all forget to take care of ourselves well. What's needed is for you to be able to honestly assess how you are caring for yourself and then to get into healthy habits of self-care. Taking good care of yourself is basic, enlightened self-interest. It is the means by which you can safely cross this huge chasm you're facing and land in a state of well-being on the other side.

What You Can Do

It's my experience that when we find ourselves dealing with a crisis, it is sometimes difficult to see the big picture because we're so focused on the crisis itself. That's one of the reasons I've included this lesson, so you can expand your horizons to include self-care along with the things you are doing for your loved one. Like the other ideas in this book, I offer the suggestions that follow with the understanding that when we're in times of darkness, we can't always easily figure what to do or how to do it. That's especially true, I believe, when it comes to the matter of self-care.

- *Breathe!* We all slip into a habit of shallow, unproductive breathing when we're under stress. Learning to control your breathing, to take good, deep breaths *especially* when you're under stress, is very important for your well-being. The quality of response that you have to offer in a crisis—in dealing with a rude hospital employee or hearing shocking news from your loved one's doctor, for instance—is going to be greatly improved by the quality of your breathing. Take a deep breath and hold it for a few beats then let it out slowly. If nothing else, this will give you a few moments to compose yourself to respond to whatever has created the crisis. Be aware of your breathing and remind yourself to breathe deeply. You'll get more oxygen than if you're doing a lot of shallow rapid breathing, and that alone will be a big help to you.

- *Exercise is a necessity.* Exercise is a good, healthy practice for a variety of reasons. For stress reduction, you need to exercise a minimum of thirty minutes *every day.* The thirty minutes does not have to be done all at once. You can divide it into smaller amounts of time—five, ten, or fifteen minutes—and duck it into your schedule throughout the day. Whatever you choose to do, make it something that appeals to you—make it fun! This is not punishment or drudgery; this is an activity you are engaging in to treat yourself well. If you approach exercise as a duty and not as a delight, then you're not going to keep it up. What do you *like* to do? Walking for half an hour every day is a wonderful way to relieve stress while exercising and enjoying the benefits of fresh air. If you can manage to take your walk through an area of beauty, how much better for your well-being! The meditative exercises such as t'ai chi chuan or yoga are another wonderful way to relieve stress. Gardening is good, meditative exercise. What about dancing? Put on some music and dance around the house. Go out in the backyard and swing a golf club, or hit tennis balls against a wall. Remember, whatever exercise you engage in is for your benefit— and enjoyment.

- *Healthy eating is another good choice.* Like exercise, eating right has lots of health benefits, along with reducing the effects of stress on your body. Food is both a source of sustenance and of pleasure. One way to honor your body for the work you're asking of it is to treat the food you put into it as both sustenance and pleasure. Make time for meals that you can savor. Reduce the number of fast food meals to nearly zero. There's little to savor, you're probably eating on the run, and most of this kind of food is full of fat, which is not good for your body. Well-balanced, nutritious, and tasty meals are not an extravagance; they're a necessity if you want to be at your best in caring for your loved one. Pay attention to the food groups you're eating—fruits and vegetables, proteins, grains, and dairy products—to do your best to ensure that you get a healthy mix, which means heavy on the fruits and vegetables and light on the fats. Remember that a healthy diet doesn't have much white stuff in it like refined sugar, white flour, and white rice. Another hallmark of a healthy diet is moderation in alcohol consumption. Don't skip meals. Be sure to eat at least three meals a day—or a half-dozen little healthy snacks. Finally, this should not be a time for austerity. Healthy eating doesn't have to be painful, and there's always room for a little comfort food, regardless of where it may fit—or not—in a recommended diet. With comfort foods, as well as alcohol and chocolate, moderation means less is better than more. Drink lots of water. No joke; just as it's important for the patient, it's important for you.

- *Use professional caregivers.* Whether you need help for just a few hours each week or with a particular task of medical caregiving, there are agencies that can provide someone to fill your particular gap. Too many caregivers burn themselves out because they erroneously believe there's no one to turn to. Nonsense! There are non-profit organizations, such as Visiting Nurses Association, to help with specific tasks, as well as agencies that can provide paid help to work with you and your loved one. The medical team or hospital social worker can help you find these sources of help. When that's not possible, try the yellow pages phone directory under *health services, health care services, home health services,* or *home care agencies.* A source of non-professional backup help can be your (or your loved one's) faith community. Members of a congregation are usually willing to set up a support service to give a primary caregiver a regular break. Taking on the task of being a caregiver isn't an invitation to martyrdom, and if you're treating it that way, then you're not truly supporting your loved one or treating yourself well. Don't be a martyr. Find a way to get some extra help so you can get a break for time to yourself, or even to get a good night's sleep.

- *Getting enough sleep is important.* How much sleep are you programming for yourself? If you are pushing back bedtime hours after you're normally in bed or getting up well before your normal waking hour in order to get to the items on your to-do list, then you aren't serving your body well. And that probably means you're not giving your loved ones your best either. Most adults require between six and eight hours of uninterrupted sleep every night. If you're not getting that and it's because of choices you're making to stay awake to get things done, you need to reprogram your list and drop off some of the items. What would you say to your patients if they were foregoing the sleep they need by trying to do too much? Well, it's time to have that same conversation with yourself, if you are reducing your sleep time to attend to your to-do list. Likewise, if caring for your loved ones and meeting their needs—or demands—is interrupting that six to eight hours of sleep you need, I strongly urge you to make use of overnight professional care for your patients. A professional or a volunteer relief caregiver can be brought in so you can get the sleep you need to maintain your health and continue to care for them. However, if your lack of sleep is involuntary, if you have the time and quiet place to sleep but stay awake in spite of your desire to sleep, then it's time to consult a doctor. Sleeplessness is sometimes a physical expression of stress. It's a process that feeds on itself with increasingly negative results. When we're not able to fall asleep or stay asleep, we can become stressed by the fact that we're awake, which only leads to less sleep. You have to judge how your inability to sleep is affecting your waking life. If you're feeling physical impacts, like lack of energy and mental confusion, give your doctor a call.

- *You need time off for yourself.* Having time away from your caregiving duties, either on your own or with friends, is another reason to use an outside agency occasionally to provide care to your loved one. It's also a good reason to set up your own support team of friends and family. Time away may be how you can get the exercise you need. It may seem an extravagance to play golf once a week with your pals when your wife is seriously ill, but doing so helped my brother-in-law, Chuck, manage the stress of caring for my sister and their teenage son. Consider taking a one- to three-day trip to a place close to home. As Dr. Kubler-Ross says, you have to treat yourself with compassion, and this is one important place to do so. Take a break from your duties as caregiver, from your job, and from your other responsibilities, not less than once a week. Time to get away from *all* of the demands on you is really important because you are looking for the light of blessings in your time of darkness. You need to step outside of that dark place on a regular basis to see where the light is at play, like stepping outside at night to see the stars scattered across the black sky. And you need to be disciplined about doing this because there are an infinite number of ways in which you can sabotage yourself by responding to the endless needs for your time to be spent on the ever-present to-do list. Make it a hard rule at first, and it will become easier to abide by later: "Every Saturday morning, I will spend two hours doing something fun, by myself if necessary, or with someone else." "On Mondays, Wednesdays, and Fridays when I come home from work, I will go into the bedroom, shut the door, and read for an hour." "I'll go to the movies every Sunday afternoon." You get the idea. This is important stress-reduction time, and you need to take it in order to be able to care for your loved one as effectively as possible.

• *Set limits on what you will do for your loved ones.* Your loved ones may be extremely dependent on you and will want you to constantly provide them with the care they feel they need. There needs to be a balance between both of your needs so you have time to attend to your own life. This is a lesson I learned from a friend who was caring for her very demanding mother. She started out responding to every request her mother made, regardless of her own needs or the actual necessity of what her mother was asking for. Soon, her mother was running her ragged, until she decided that it would be all right to not answer each and every one of her mother's demands on an immediate basis. She worked out a schedule with her mother that allowed her to have some downtime, and her mother eventually came to accept that her requests would be met on the agreed-upon schedule, not when the idea occurred to her.

• *Have your own team to support you.* I have a group of female friends who were so important to my well-being when my sister was sick. They are close friends with whom I can share my feelings—they provided a safe haven where I could vent. In addition, being with them was one of the ways I could get regular breaks. We'd get together for dinner or other outings. They also telephoned occasionally between our get-togethers. These check-in calls were helpful because I was reminded of the presence of the safety net that these women provided me. Don't forget about banking offers of help that I mentioned in Lesson Seven. Creating their own support team is a hard concept for most caregivers to accept because they are so focused on *giving* care that they don't realize the extent to which they need to *receive* care themselves. One of the greatest gifts you can give yourself is to create your own team, just as you are a member of the patient's team. You may have more than one—perhaps one group at work and one group from some other area of your life. These are the people with whom you can talk and share your feelings. They can also be the ones who help you take your breaks, who are your exercise buddies, or who will go on some little excursion or outing with you and *not* talk about your loved one's medical problems, if that's what you need. Like my friends were for me, this group is *your* circle, the people who come together to support you in whatever way you may need.

- *Find a way to express your feelings.* There are lots of ways to let those feelings out, especially the so-called negative feelings of anger, resentment, and betrayal. ("What betrayal? I don't feel betrayed. Well, maybe just a little bit since we won't be doing—fill in the blank—because of the medical crisis.") I don't believe it's necessary to label those feelings as negative or positive, good or bad. They are simply your feelings, and all of your feelings need to be brought out into the open so they don't start causing your body problems. Think of feelings as a whole bunch of rambunctious Great Dane- or St. Bernard-sized puppies that want to come outside to play. If they're playing inside, they create a chaos of overturned furniture, torn curtains and pillows, shredded house plants, and broken vases and lamps. But let them outdoors where they can run and bark and play without wrecking the furniture, and all the energy goes into a place that has room for it. So let the puppies out by journaling or using some other creative form of expression. One of my favorites is to write a letter to God. I'll confess that at first it's a bit daunting to be expressing anger to God, but I've discovered that he can take it and is willing to support me while I get the anger and its underlying fear out of its hiding place. The need to share feelings is one of the primary reasons that support groups exist, and if you have access to one, I highly recommend that you investigate joining it. Sharing your feelings is one of the reasons to create your own support team because there will be things you want to say that you won't feel comfortable saying to your loved ones. That doesn't lessen the necessity of sharing your feelings with them too. The idea of journaling or a support group is to be able to let the puppies out in their most energetic form and let them get to know how they play. Then, one at a time, as an appropriate opportunity presents itself, you can take them and share them with your patient. If you're fearful that your loved one isn't going to survive the illness, you need to be able to talk about that together. There may be fears he or she wants to share with you too. Nobody benefits when feelings go unexpressed.

- *Prioritize and limit your to-do list.* This can't be said often enough—let go of some of your responsibilities and put others that you keep lower on the priority list. Let go of the small stuff. Keeping the house white-glove clean or staying on the board of a volunteer organization isn't as important as what you are doing for your loved one, so be willing to establish priorities and let go of the items that aren't as important for the time being. You have taken on an enormous assignment if you're caring for a loved one. No one should expect you to do so *and* maintain all your other responsibilities. Prioritizing your activities will require you to actually create a list of all the things that you do every day. You will probably be surprised by how lengthy the list is. Include everything you do for yourself, your family, your employer, and anyone else you have a responsibility to—church groups, schools groups, youth groups, community organizations, political organizations, or whatever it is. The next step is to decide which activities or responsibilities to keep and which to cut back on so you have new time in your daily rounds to spend in giving care. The hard part will be to stick to the new to-do list and not fall back to the old one. It's especially hard when friends or colleagues insist that they can't get along without you. Cultivate the thought—and practice saying it—that yes, they can get along without you. The PTA, Cub Scouts, church group, political activities, investment club, or whatever it is got along without you once, and they can do so again. Even if you're the founding power behind something, it's probably time for the organization to grow beyond you and discover how it can operate without your presence. Cut out some activities and reduce your involvement in others. Believe me, the world will be full of opportunities to re-involve yourself when your time of being a caregiver is over.

- *Get whatever training you need.* Providing some degree of medical care to your loved one at home is a huge source of stress. Obviously, if you're going to have to provide this care, you're going to have to learn new skills, whether it's from the Internet, from a member of the medical team, or from the patient. Make time to learn whatever is needed so you can provide the care with relaxed confidence. A good source of training resources can be the social worker or ombudsman at the hospital where your loved one is being treated. Don't be deterred by a medical team that doesn't have the time or the personnel to train you. Gently but firmly insist that they make the time to teach you what you need to learn, or find another source for the training you want. Don't take no for an answer when you're seeking training to care for your loved one. The only way I know of to remove the stress from providing the medical care your loved one needs is to become proficient at whatever those particular skills are.

- *Manage your stress at work.* Since a job by itself can be a huge source of stress, now is the time to find ways to keep the job stress at a manageable level. If your job requires regular breaks, take them; don't work through *any* of your breaks. *Always* take your lunch break away from your work station. Go to the lunch room, take your lunch outside, or take a walk during your lunch break. Do something recreational during your lunch hour—a game of chess, a card game, or team sport. Read a book. Go shopping, if that's feasible. You don't have to buy anything; just looking can be a relaxing and enjoyable experience. Decide whether working additional hours for the bigger paycheck is more important than reducing hours for time with your loved one. When there's a financial impact from the medical condition, this can be a pressure-laden choice. When you've made those decisions, create a job plan and stick to it. Learn to set limits on what you will take on in terms of work. This isn't easy to do. My experience has been that work expands to fit the willingness of someone to do it—there will always be more work to do than you have time for. Especially if you've opted to reduce work time to care for your loved one, you need to be confident in saying no to additional assignments in order to have the time and energy to devote to your caregiving. Make use of any support systems your employer offers, such as Employee Assistance Programs (EAPs) or in-house peer counseling or support groups. If those aren't available, cultivate your own on-the-job support team of fellow workers with whom you can talk about your experiences of caring for your loved one.

- *Find a source for emotional/psychological help.* Whether you find this through your work or whether it's through referral of your physician or the patient's medical team, the use of outside counseling or support groups is important to your well-being, just as it is for the patient's. Too often caregivers assume they shouldn't seek help because it is their loved ones, not they, who are in a serious condition. You may need help in order to stay healthy, physically and emotionally, so you can continue to support and care for the patient. Denying that you're having trouble when you're feeling helpless and hopeless isn't going to benefit you or your loved ones.

- *Slow down.* One of the reasons to reorder your priorities is to provide you with more time to be with your

loved ones. There are varying qualities of time, however, so that time just by itself may not be what you or
they need. Approaching your time with your patients
on a constantly restricted schedule—"I've got to be out
of here, in my car, and on the street in five minutes"—
is clearly not beneficial for them or you. Slow down.
Reprioritizing your life is about creating a higher quality of time to spend with the patient and with yourself.
Don't run through your life, walk through it, and stop
frequently to examine and admire what you see. It's
one of the reasons to give yourself regular treats. We
are physical creatures, and we live in a physical realm.
Constant rushing creates stress. God has given us a
beautiful world, full of wondrous things that we are
here to learn from, if we'll just slow down enough to
do so. It's one of the great blessings of this time in your
life—learning to slow down, to be genuinely present
not just to the patient but to yourself as well. One way
to do this is to create decompression time between your
outside responsibilities and your time with your loved
one. When you get home from work, take a five- to
fifteen-minute break alone to unwind from your outer
routine and to get into the rhythm of the patient's routine. Likewise, you may want to decompress from long
periods spent with the patient, in order to shift gears
into what you'll be doing next. Snooze, read, journal,
meditate, look at a magazine, stare at the ceiling, and
listen to music. All of these are good ways to make
those mental shifts so you can be fully present in whatever part of your life you're functioning in.

- *Give yourself regular treats.* This is a bit different from
taking a break, although it is certainly part of it. Com-

fort food is a treat. Renting movies you love is a treat. Listening to—and singing along with—favorite music in your car is a treat. Reading a magazine on a hobby or interest of yours is a treat. Watching or going to a ball game (any kind of ball game) is a treat. Having lighted candles on the dinner table is a treat. Calling a friend long distance to talk without worrying about the time is a treat. Taking a long bath—perhaps with bubbles—is a treat. What little things can you do to pamper yourself? No doubt you're doing what you can to provide simple pleasures for your loved one. What are you doing to provide the same nurturing for yourself?

- *Make time to read and learn.* This is another gift of time. Obviously, you have been learning a lot about medicine and your loved one's condition, and that's important. But ask yourself what else you would like to learn. One of the blessings you can discover is that there are soul lessons in this time, some from your direct experience and some from the wisdom of others. Reading good books or magazines is one way to access this wisdom. You may also learn about yourself and about what your interests and passions truly are. Try not to limit yourself by restricting what you read or learn from to those things you need for your job or even for your role as caregiver. Let your mind be free to point you in a new direction without being restricted to things that should be read. What kinds of things interest you? Pick up a magazine or a book on that subject and then be willing to see where that leads you.

- *Make time for spiritual growth and expression.* This is a great gift to give yourself during this time of darkness.

Remember that God is intimately present in this process for both you and your loved one. Make time to draw closer to the divine. Consider it a directed search for light. There are a number of ways to accomplish this—from meditation and prayer to keeping a prayer journal (to record your conversations with God and the insights that result), to joining a study group or even going on retreat if you can manage to take the time away. Retreats for caregivers are becoming more and more prevalent. Look for them through various faith communities or through your loved one's local disease support organization. Receiving spiritual counseling from a person of faith—a monk, priest, imam, nun, prayer leader, or minister—can be a way to make this a time of spiritual enlargement. There are probably hundreds of thousands of books on spiritual subjects that you can read. Journaling, either as a means of following your prayer life or just as a basic means of expressing your feelings, is an excellent way to track your spiritual responses to caring for your loved one. There are great soul-level rewards to be gained if you can find the patience to listen for them when they are presented to you.

- *Enjoy intimacy and love.* This is another practice that you may find difficult to incorporate into your daily round because you are so focused on *giving* that it may be hard to shift into a mode of *receiving*. That's really what this is about, allowing yourself to receive intimacy—either physical or emotional—and affection. One reason it may be so difficult to accept love from others is that you've gone into a defensive mode, shutting down your feelings in order not to have to deal with highly-charged emotions during this difficult time. You've pulled up your drawbridge and are safely ensconced behind your castle walls where no one can enter with bad—or good—news. But you're locked in there with all those destructive puppies that need to be let out, and there are people outside who have plenty of love to offer you. You really need to put the bridge back down so you can let your feelings out and invite the waiting love in. My husband, Paul, was my rock during my sister's illness, constantly offering me his love and support in a variety of ways. Yes, the physical act of lovemaking was part of what he gave me, but so was a willingness to listen, as much as he could, to what was happening with the progress of MaryKay's illness. And most important, he literally was the shoulder that I cried on. Don't fall into the trap of being such a source of strength for everyone else that you don't acknowledge your own need to be loved and strengthened by those around you. If you're caring for your spouse, who can you turn to for the intimacy of shared thoughts and feelings? Siblings, parents, children, and close friends all can provide the love that you need, just as you're providing it for the patient.

• *Play, have fun, and laugh.* This is also a hard one to understand and practice. You may not see much to laugh about with your loved one's medical circumstance, and you may feel that play, fun, or enjoyment are not appropriate given your loved one's serious condition. Remember Norman Cousins's experience about the healing nature of fun and laughter, how it helps set up a hopeful and positive attitude that's necessary to well-being. Don't forget the e-mail request for jokes sent out by my cousin and his wife. There is just as great a necessity for you to utilize the medicine of laughter as there is for the patient. Read the funnies in the newspaper. Take in a comedy at the movies. Find a humorous book at the library and read it. Do something on a regular basis that allows you to experience and enjoy silliness and play. You can incorporate play in your time for exercise and/or when you take breaks. Have you skipped anywhere in recent memory? Do you even remember how? Can you still whistle a tune? Singing is a great way to play. Discover the joy of being in your body, of having fun.

Please regard all of the suggestions on this list as a starting point to which you can bring your own creative approach to the matter of caring for yourself, just as you are using your creativity to care for your loved one. I want to acknowledge the importance of what you are doing in providing this loving care. You are living out love and compassion, the highest gifts that we can offer one another because they echo the gifts of love and mercy that God graces us with each moment. As you provide the love, support, and care that your loved one needs, learn to love, support, and care for yourself at the same time. This gift to yourself will enable you to carry out your chosen assignment to the best of your ability, and it will be one of the ways to discover blessings for yourself in your time of darkness.

CONCLUSION:
LIFE IS MESSY

August 1, 1999, Mammoth Lakes, California

A lake, even the smallest one, can never be completely known from just one place on the shore, because your understanding of it is limited to what you can see from a given perspective. At Lake McCleoud, if you stand on the eastern shore, you understand the lake as a basin anchored beneath huge granite cliffs, a place that captures snowmelt from the peaks above. But if you stand on the shore beneath those cliffs, then you know the lake as hanging on the edge of a precipice that drops to Long Valley and feeds all the lakes below it. You have to walk all the way around it, or climb up the cliff above it, to see its totality—to know what the lake is in all its aspects. It's the same with big events in my life, especially the experiences of the past year. I'm a ways from walking all the way around them, so I don't have the complete view yet.

Human beings—all of us, no matter how saintly—innately want to control most, if not all, aspects of our lives. It's an urge we're born with. When they are not sleeping, babies do nothing but work at controlling the world that surrounds them, fussing, crying, or outright screaming to get those large beings around them to do what they want: clean me up, let me sleep, entertain me, feed me, and feed me *now*. Our developmental stages revolve around learning to accept what we can and cannot control. By the time we reach our middle adult years, at least by age forty, most of us realize the list of things we can control is limited to what we do, think, and feel, and the list of what we can't control—which is everything else in life—is very long indeed. But that doesn't mean that inside each of us there still isn't that being we were born into who still wants life to be a controllable vision of perfection, with all details resolved to a tidy Hollywood-style ending in which the bad, those who won't be controlled, are killed off or at least severely punished and the good and heroic, us, live happily ever after.

From your perspective right now, life must look pretty uncontrollable. There are no carefully orchestrated fadeouts as you and your loved one ride off into the sunset. Instead, what you've got are a lot of factors beyond your control, from the medical condition of your loved ones to the treatments they are receiving and their cost, to your patients' reaction to the disease and treatments, and to their response to the care you're providing. Not only is it not tidy, it's downright messy. That's part of the darkness—the realization that none of these circumstances may come out the way you want them to.

Your loved one may survive the medical crisis, but his or her life and yours will be changed forever. The injury will be permanently disabling, the illness will be chronic, the disease will be in remission but the treatments will have had a lasting physical impact, or the condition will have forced a significant change in lifestyle. If the condition is terminal, you are facing the reality of living on without your loved one. In your vision of a perfect world, losing him or her this way, at this point in your life, was probably something you didn't envision—it was never a part of your plan for your life.

A medical crisis is a great teacher of many lessons, the most basic being that life is not neat and tidy. It's often downright messy. On just about any level you can imagine, a serious illness or injury shows us that life isn't about precision. Dealing with treatments and side effects; medications and medical equipment—sometimes intruding into your living room; insurance companies and hospitals; medical people and the responses of friends and family, all demonstrate over and over again that life can be physically messy.

As you and your patients try to assimilate information about what's happening, you've discovered that for every article you read about a given treatment for their condition, there is another article that is equally well researched that advocates something else. The causes of some diseases are still not fully understood, and as a result, the cures are open to often-heated debate. By now, you've no doubt realized that there is no one single way to approach their treatment. The rational, scientific method of traditional medicine is still as much art as it is science, and that's not as neat and tidy as we have been used to thinking that it is. Sometimes two plus two just won't add up to four.

If you're paying attention, the lesson is repeated on deeper levels as well. The spiritual questions you're encountering are deep and numerous. There is something important—acceptance—to be learned in the fact that there are no answers, particularly not to the why. It's a mystery, and one that you can't solve. In learning acceptance of your loved one's state of being, and your own, you allow yourself a wonderful opportunity to encounter life in a new way.

Physician/author Susan Kuner, writing of her post-breast

cancer experiences in *Speak the Language of Healing*, talks about her altered ground of being, in which "the tenor of [her] mind, the texture of [her] heart" has fundamentally changed. The conclusion for her, and for you, is inescapable: life is messy but can be meaningful if we are able to move beyond our very human need to do and thus somehow control it. Life reaches a higher plane when we can drop "doing" in order to achieve a state of being. Dr. Kuner now has a list of essentials for living, which include spending more time with family and friends, hanging out with lots of children, sticking to what is real, acting with courage, standing on the ground of simplicity, and, perhaps most important of all, cherishing this precious gift of life.[1]

The Blessing of Acceptance

This messiness of life can be a blessing in this time of darkness, if you can truly come to embrace and accept the understanding that, along with the imprecision, meaning is also present. That sounds a bit absurd, doesn't it? But the truth of it is that when we can learn to release that innate desire to control things outside of ourselves—when we quit trying to fix things—we are at a point that allows us to look for and embrace the purpose of our lives. And that process then allows us to accept the people we love, with the understanding that their lives have a special meaning too. Psychiatrist and teacher Elisabeth Kubler-Ross outlines this process:

> In working with the dying and the living, it becomes clear that most of us are challenged by the same lessons: the lesson of fear, the lesson of guilt, the lesson of anger, the lesson of forgiveness, the lesson of surrender, the lesson of time, the lesson of patience, the lesson of love, the lesson of rela-

tionships, the lesson of play, the lesson of loss, the lesson of power, the lesson of authenticity, and the lesson of happiness. Learning lessons is a little like reaching maturity. You're not suddenly more happy, wealthy, or powerful, but you understand the world around you better, and you're at peace with yourself.[2]

Recall the story of Ané and my sister in Lesson Eight, "Being with the Patient," and how Ané was bothered by MaryKay's shopping habits. Ané learned—in dealing with her negative response to MK's desire to go shopping—how to accept MaryKay and her shopping trips. Even more important than Ané's acceptance of my sister's personal quirks is the fact that Ané has carried that release of control into other relationships. That has become a *big* blessing to her and the other people in her life. In learning this lesson, Ané was clear about what her feelings were; she has limits on what she'll buy and when she'll go shopping, but she was also able to let go of the outcome—MaryKay's need to go shopping.

Once again, this is a lesson about *being* and not *doing*. When we're in a state of *being*, we're not trying to control things. *Doing* frequently brings with it attempts to control the other forces and factors in our lives that we simply cannot control. While the example of Ané and MaryKay may seem frivolous, I offer it as an easily understood living example of twin principles: the need to know your truth and the need to let go of the outcome when it involves others. The world's great religions and spiritual practices incorporate this principle because it allows the person who can learn this lesson to be at peace by not struggling against the divine plan—however messy or chaotic it may appear to be in our human frame of reference:

- Taoism teaches acceptance of the essential nature of things—simple living and the acceptance of the flow of life. "The ancient saying, 'Surrender brings perfection' is not just empty words. Truly, to the yielding comes the perfect; to the perfect comes the whole universe" (Tao Te Ching, Verse 22).

- Buddhism teaches that life (a separated existence) brings suffering, that suffering has its roots in desires, and that by destroying desire—we might say desire to control—unity with the universe, or Nirvana, can be reached. "And what have I taught? I have taught that suffering exists, that suffering has an origin, that suffering has an end. Why have I taught this? Because this is useful, it has to do with real Truth. It leads to the cessation of passion, it brings peace, supreme wisdom, the holy life, and Nirvana" (The Buddha, "My Teachings").

- Judeo-Christian tradition is based on a fundamental call to be obedient to God and, in that obedience, to put aside the self's need to make choices or to control the forces of life. "He gives strength to the weary and increases the power of the weak. Even youths grow tired and weary, and young men stumble and fall; but those who hope in the Lord will renew their strength. They will soar on wings like eagles; they will run and not grow weary, they will walk and not be faint" (Isaiah 40:29–31).

- Christ himself warns that this lesson is hard to learn because we keep wanting to make ourselves the arbiters of what's peaceful. But he also reminds us that acceptance enables us to be free of fear. "Peace I leave with you; my peace I give to you. I do not give to you as the world gives. Do not let your hearts be troubled, and do not let them be afraid" (John 14:27 NRSV)

- The Bhagavad Gita, the "Song of God" in the Hindu tradition, is a poetic story of the archer Arjuna. It records his coming to understand how his illusions about the true nature of the world prevented him from seeing the true nature of Krishna, the Lord of the Universe. The poem ends as Arjuna surrenders his will to Krishna. "O Krishna, through your grace the foe of delusion has been destroyed; the clear light of wisdom has dawned … O Lord, I stand here, ready, to do as you command" (The Bhagavad Gita, Chapter 18).

- The Sufi poets of Islam write of their desire to merge with God, the Beloved. They focus on the necessity to release their individuality and to accept the world as it is in order to know the Beloved. "Every particle of creation sings its own song of what is, and of what is not. The wise hear what is; the mad hear what is not—and only a cracked mirror will show a difference" (Ghalib).

(All of the foregoing, with the exception of the quotation from the book of Isaiah and the gospel of John, came from *The Inner Treasure: An Introduction to the World's Sacred and Mystical Writings,* by Jonathan Star, who translated all of the texts.)

The late Cardinal Joseph Bernardin, the Archbishop of Chicago, was a beloved and respected leader of the contemporary Catholic Church in the United States, who recorded his thoughts and feelings as he was dying of pancreatic cancer. His book, *The Gift of Peace,* resounds with this principle of surrender:

> The more we cling to ourselves and others, the more we try to control our destiny—the more we lose the true sense of our lives, the more we are impacted by the futility of it all. It's precisely in letting go, in entering into complete union with the Lord, in letting him take over, that we discover our

true selves. It's in the act of abandonment that we experience redemption, that we find life, peace, and joy in the midst of physical, emotional, and spiritual suffering.[3]

Giving Care as an Expression of Love

Another of the lessons that I've learned is that the gifts I've received from caring for an ill friend or family member have come to me *regardless of the outcome*. I must confess that it was a lesson that wasn't readily apparent when my mother was ill and dying because I wanted her to not be ill and to not die. Obviously, my attempts to control her medical outcome produced nothing but frustration and anguish for me. Why was this happening to her—and to me—were the constant questions I threw at God in my prayers, alternating with pleas that God grant us a miracle and cure her. Later, I pleaded with God to take her quickly and painlessly so she wouldn't have to suffer so much.

It wasn't until the moment of her death, when I was witness to the departure of her soul from her body, that I began to perceive that I'd been granted a profound privilege in caring for her and in being present as she was born into the next life. In that moment, I began to understand that all of us who cared for Mom were given an opportunity to physically express our love for her in the time we spent together.

My family is not one that frequently shared expressions of affection, beyond a quick hug and an occasionally spoken "I love you." The shift that occurred in her illness was that in giving her our caring and support, we were allowed to move beyond our usual mode of expressing our love for one another. We now had a new language of giving and receiving love through the shared experience of a serious illness, in finding the light in the darkness together, and in being allowed to express this deep affection in caregiving. You too have a rare and wondrous privilege to translate your love into a physical action, whether it is in active caregiving or just being with your loved one.

What, exactly, are these gifts of love that flow through your caregiving? I think there are four:

- *Your presence*—Serious illness or injury can be a horrifically isolating experience. And yet our highest calling as both human and spiritual beings is to love one another, to connect to others, and to remove the barriers of isolation. Anyone who has experienced a life-threatening condition knows that friends and family can remain distant, out of an inability—or unwillingness—to confront their own mortality by being witness to someone else's journey to the edge of life. Again and again, I have seen the sorrow of patients over the absence of friends or even family at this tremendously important stage of their lives. Your great gift of love is to remain close to your friends or family members. By being part of a group, or even being the sole individual who provides them with physical care, you are also providing them with emotional sustenance, which is as important to them in this time as are the treatments they are receiving. This is not an easy gift to present, nor is it inevitably easy for them to receive. You both have your emotional stages to work through, and the life changes wrought by the illness are hard on everybody. Your ability to express your love for them and their ability to accept it are going to be colored by a lifetime of experiences and by the behaviors that have been shaped by those experiences. And yet you *are* with them, caring for them, supporting them, providing loving company on this medical journey they find themselves undertaking. It is a great gift for them to be saved from soul-killing isolation and for you to have a means to express your love in caring for them.

- *Healing*—As I have pointed out earlier, there is a significant difference between cure and healing. Cure is the restoration of the body to its state of health; healing is a restoration of the self to its wholeness. It is possible to have healing in the end stages of a life because healing is an internal process, the work of the heart and soul, as opposed to being the work of the physical body, although it is possible to integrate the two. The benefits of this inner restoration can come to you, the caregiver, as well as to the patient. In fact, your presence in the medical process of your loved one can often lead to a joint participation in healing by you both. Healing involves the release of regrets; the recognition of old injuries, both those received and those you've given; and reconciliation or forgiveness of those past wounding experiences. It's a process that's best served by interaction between patients and the people who are significant in their lives. As a caregiver, your gift can be to help facilitate these moments and to participate yourself when you and the patient have a relationship that needs restoring in some way.

- *Confronting mortality*—This is another gift that as a caregiver you can both give and receive. We are, after all, mortal creatures. We all will die at some point in time. Living with that understanding can be very freeing, yet so many people live in ways designed, either consciously or unconsciously, to avoid this very fundamental fact. Human beings can become so attached to this physical life and so fearful of what comes after it that they cling to the purely physical in order to avoid having to confront the fact that this existence will end. We fill up our lives with things to do, with material objects, or with attempts to turn back the clock by making ourselves look younger. But none of it matters because our lives *will* end, whether we want them to or not. Only when we're able to accept the reality of our own deaths can we live fully, genuinely, and authentically. It's the state of peace or being that the great religions describe. Remember Rabbi Ben Kamin's principle that a breath of death yields a good swallow of life. You are giving this gift as you work through your process of the five stages, when you can be attuned to the patient's process as well, and most especially if you and your loved one can talk about the process and share your thoughts and feelings about it. I believe that this particular gift, like healing, is experienced both as a process and also in reflecting together on what the process feels like.

Regardless of the outcome of your loved one's condition, sharing these gifts can create profound changes for both of you. With your presence, in the way in which you share in your loved one's healing, and with acceptance of mortality, you both will find yourselves in that *new ground of being,* described by Dr. Kuner, with a new "tenor of mind and texture of heart." This new place can be exciting, motivational to others, and continuously inspirational. It's a state of being even in the midst of doing, and it brings with it some very profound, life-changing discoveries:

- Life slows to a more deliberate pace in which you are able to be fully present to *all* that surrounds you.

- You use a new yardstick for measuring what's important and what's not worthy of the precious time that you've been given.

- You have less tolerance for the artificial and a greater need for what is genuine and true.

When you begin living your life in this way, you may even find that longstanding ideas and relationships are not as you want them to be. To think about changing—or ending—relationships that have endured over time may seem frightening, if not downright bizarre. But when you have reached the understanding of your mortality and the valuable gift of your time in life, then these reassessments—and the changes that sometimes result from them—are far easier to contemplate than ever before.

When living an authentic life becomes your goal, reassessments and significant changes are the inevitable result. You may discover that your job has become simply so much work and that you know you have a vocation elsewhere that you are determined to discover. Reaching that conclusion and then taking the steps to move into something new is not easy. Getting out of the old job and into whatever needs to come next may be complex and difficult, but the decision to make the change and the drive to see it through will come from a new awareness that will take the sting out of the process.

What Are You Going To Do?

I've concluded each of the preceding section's chapters with a list of ideas entitled "What You Can Do." Now it's time for you to ask yourself: What am I going to do with the lessons I've been learning? What have I learned from the light of blessings that have come to me in this time of darkness?

For many, it's back to life as it was before the medical crisis. They will imagine the lessons were restricted to information, facts, and tips about how to deal with medical teams and hospitals and insurance companies and where to get good medical information at the local library or on the Internet. If that's what they've learned, then life will definitely be unchanged for them, except for whatever physical changes have resulted from their loved one's illness or injury. Are you going to be one of those who let the blessings fall around them but don't bother to pick them up and incorporate them into their life? I hope not.

The lessons you've learned—or are learning—as a result of your loved one's condition won't necessarily be offered to you just once. Margaret, my therapist, likens life to a trip on a winding road that circles up a mountain. In traveling this road around and around the mountain, you will come back to the same view over and over again. The thing to remember is that if you're learning, if you're progressing up the mountain toward the summit, then the view gets a little wider each time you circle because you're a bit higher up on the mountain each time you come to it. That's what the light is for, an opportunity for each of us to see a little more—to understand a little better—what our lives are for and about. The blessings and lessons are the ways in which we enlarge our perspective as we travel this climbing road.

So what do you propose to do with this new perspective that you're acquiring? Mike, the friend who was nearly paralyzed in an automobile accident, worked very, very hard to recover the use of his legs. But he didn't let the process stop there. Once an executive with a huge multinational corporation, he has become a powerful motivational speaker. Mike now inspires others, both injured and uninjured, to take life as the great gift that it is and overcome whatever barriers they face in order to live in fully meaningful ways.

Ané de Nio, who actively cared for my sister, has found a vocation in assisting people who are facing a medical crisis. She took three weeks to live with a friend who was suffering from cancer. Ané cared for her friend's children while the friend recovered from the effects of chemotherapy. After that, she "adopted" a nursing home patient who had no family. She visited him regularly until he died a little more than a year later.

Now in remission from her cancer, my sister-in-law, Rosemarie, and her husband, Bob, reprioritized their lives. They moved to a new home that allowed them to be closer to the things they loved to do, and Bob set in motion plans to retire from his own business. They travel now, something they had been putting off until "later." Rosemarie created a list of events to attend and places to visit—including the Kentucky Derby—and she and Bob have been systematically taking those trips, a way of recognizing the gift of time she's been given.

Do these changes occur overnight? The best ones probably don't. It takes time and quiet to come to an understanding of what the lessons have been and how they need to play out in your life.

Tom, the man who nearly lost himself in providing non-stop care for his wife, Beverly, told me after her death that it took him a long time to realize what had happened to his own life. Once he had that realization, he decided to take a year to himself, to contemplate what meaning there was in his experiences with Beverly and to decide what to do next.

In caring for your loved one, you have gained wisdom of all

kinds—practical, spiritual, and emotional. While you're contemplating the changes that this new wisdom may make in your life, bear in mind that one gift you can give to others is to share what you've learned, as I am sharing my lessons with you. You may by nature be a teacher, so talking to someone else about your experiences will come naturally.

On the other hand, if you're not so inclined, there are still ways in which you can share what you've learned, just by having a simple conversation with someone or writing out a few ideas that you felt were most helpful and then sharing those notes. One of the great sources of light that comes from a support group is this sharing of information and experiences. It's a torch that we pass on to one another. I hope you will continue to do so, so others who find themselves in the darkness will be able to benefit from the light of blessings you have received. Sharing what you've learned in order to help someone else is one of the most loving things you can do for another person, a gift that comes from your highest self.

If you choose to really live your life in a new way based on the lessons you've learned from this time of darkness, then your life *will* look different. One benefit can be to continue the self-care habits that you needed to learn in order to be able to care for your patients. Just because there's no medical crisis, it doesn't mean that you don't need to continue to follow those same "self-indulgent," healthy practices. We are physical beings, and we need to keep our bodies in good working order, just as we tend to our automobiles or even our lawn mowers.

Don't forget those particular lessons of self-care or the lessons of *being* when you are with another person. It is so easy to slip back into the old routine of hurried, busy lives and the stress they engender. While you make room in your life for self-care and support of your loved one, hold on to the principles of being rather than constantly doing. You will find your life will continue to be emotionally healthier if you can continue to remember these rules:

- Know your truth, speak it without blame or shame, and then let go of the outcome.

- Maintain the habit of active listening.

- Release regrets.

- Forgive others. And forgive yourself.

- Learn to give and receive love without reservation or without trying to protect yourself from old wounds.

Life after caregiving needs to incorporate spiritual well-being too. In sharing your loved one's encounter with mortality, you have been given a great blessing—the opportunity to move into a closer relationship with God by discovering the true meaning of life in general, and your life in particular. I hope that you have learned, as I did—and as did all of the people whose stories are a part of this book—that God is *always* present in our lives but that the divine is surely most accessible in suffering and healing.

As human beings, we are creatures of the dark, constantly seeking the light of the divine. When all is going smoothly in life—as *we* have it planned—we can convince ourselves that there is no darkness. The blessing of the medical crisis that you are confronting is that your illusion of light has been removed. There is darkness all around you, and you can't escape it. The blessing that also comes with the darkness itself is that God's light *is* there to be found. Like the darkness, the true light is all around you, if you will just seek it out.

Is the mystery of the source of your loved one's condition darkness or light? As long as you struggle with that question, as long as you try to find the answer to that ultimate mystery, your life will look very dark indeed. However, when you can accept your loved one's condition—and the mystery of why it has happened—then you can make the space in your life to surrender ultimate control to the Creator. And in that, my friend, there is nothing but the bright light and blessing of God's presence.

ENDNOTES

Lesson One: Finding the Blessings

1. Charles Yale Harrison, *Thank God for My Heart Attack*, (New York: Henry Holt & Co., 1949), 75.

2. Rabbi Ben Kamin, *The Path of the Soul: Making Peace with Mortality*, (New York: A Plume Book, 1999), 106.

3. Richard Schultz, PhD, and Scott R. Beach, PhD, Abstract: "Caregiving as a Risk Factor for Mortality: The Caregiver Health Effects Study," Journal of the American Medical Association, December, 1999, 282:2215–2219.

4. Bernie S. Siegel, MD, Introduction to *Love, Medicine and Miracles*, (New York: Harper Perennial, 1986), viii.

5. Henri Nouwen, *Seeds of Hope: A Henri Nouwen Reader*, ed. Robert Durback, (New York: Image Books/Doubleday, 1997), 86.

6. Wayne W. Dyer, *Wisdom of the Ages: 60 Days to Enlightenment*, (New York: Harper Collins, 1998), 47.

Lesson Two: The Emotional Impact

1. Elisabeth Kubler-Ross, MD, and David Kessler, *Life Lessons* (New York: Scribner, 2000), 79.

2. M. Scott Peck, MD, *Denial of the Soul: Spiritual and Medical Perspectives on Euthanasia and Mortality*, (New York: Harmony Books, 1997), 166.

3. Kubler-Ross, *Life Lessons*, 78.

4. Elisabeth Kubler-Ross, MD, *On Death and Dying,* (New York: Touchstone Books/Simon & Schuster, 1969), 147.

5. Kamin, *Denial of the Soul,* 163.

6. Kubler-Ross, *On Death and Dying,* 52.

7. Kubler-Ross, *Life Lessons,* 87.

8. Kubler-Ross, *On Death and Dying,* 53.

9. Kubler-Ross, *On Death and Dying,* 65–66.

10. Kubler-Ross, *Life Lessons,* 147.

11. Kubler-Ross, *Life Lessons,* 155.

12. Mary Susan Herczog, "A Battle with Breast Cancer," *Los Angeles Times,* December 8, 1997, Health Section, Orange County edition.

13. Kubler-Ross, *On Death and Dying,* 99.

14. Selma Schimmel and Barry Fox, *Cancer Talk,* (New York: Broadway Books, 1999), 82.

15. Dale Matthews, MD, and Connie Clark, *The Faith Factor: Proof of the Healing Power of Prayer,* (New York: Penguin Books, 1998), 148.

16. Siegel, *Love, Medicine and Miracles,* 43.

17. Kubler-Ross, *On Death and Dying,* 148–149.

18. Siegel, *Love, Medicine and Miracles,* 28.

19. Schimmel, *Cancer Talk,* 19.

Lesson Three: The Connection of Mind, Body, and Spirit

1. *The American Heritage Dictionary of the English Language, New College Edition,* ed. William Morris, (Boston: Houghton Mifflin, 1979), 1,305.

2. Siegel, Introduction to *Love, Medicine and Miracles*, ix.

3. *The American Heritage Dictionary of the English Language*, 834.

4. *The American Heritage Dictionary of the English Language*, 1,245.

5. Siegel, *Love, Medicine and Miracles*, 65.

6. R. R. Palmer and Joel Colton, *A History of the Modern World*, (New York: Alfred A. Knopf, 1965), 265.

7. Palmer, *A History of the Modern World*, 264.

8. Larry Dossey, MD, *Healing Words: The Power of Prayer and the Practice of Medicine*, (New York: Harper Paperbacks, 1993), 54–55.

9. Dossey, *Healing Words*, 55–60.

10. Matthews, *The Faith Factor*, 17.

11. Siegel, *Love, Medicine and Miracles*, 69.

12. Dyer, *Wisdom of the Ages*, 159.

13. Dyer, *Wisdom of the Ages*, 158.

14. Dyer, *Wisdom of the Ages*, 209.

15. Dyer, *Wisdom of the Ages*, 160.

16. Andrew Weil, MD, *Sound Body, Sound Mind: Music for Healing*, (Los Angeles: Rhino Recordings/Wea, 2005), 17.

17. Dossey, Introduction to *Healing Words*, xxiii.

18. Norman Cousins, *Anatomy of an Illness, as Perceived by the Patient*, (New York: W. W. Norton & Company, 1979), 18.

19. Cousins, *Anatomy of an Illness*, 18.

20. Cousins, *Anatomy of an Illness*, 18.

21. Cousins, *Anatomy of an Illness,* 40.

22. Dyer, *Wisdom of the Ages,* 176.

23. Dossey, Introduction to *Healing Words,* xxii.

Lesson Four: The Diagnosis

1. Mary Susan Herczog, "Inside the Healing Circle," *Los Angeles Times,* February 9, 1998, Health Section, Orange County edition.

2. Laura Landro, "Be Your Own Greatest Ally in Battling Cancer," *Los Angeles Times,* November 2, 1998, Health Section, Orange County edition.

3. Schimmel, *Cancer Talk,* 25.

4. Rachel Remens, MD, *Kitchen Table Wisdom: Stories That Heal,* (New York: Riverhead Books, 1996), 67.

5. Jay Antenen, "The Touch That Heals," *Cincinnati CityBeat,* July 14–20, 2004, p. 16.

6. Mary Susan Herczog, "The Who, What and Why Behind Her Treatment," *Los Angeles Times,* July 13, 1998, Health Section, Orange County edition.

7. Schimmel, *Cancer Talk,* 78.

8. Schimmel, *Cancer Talk,* 78.

9. Dossey, *Healing Words,* 48.

10. Herczog, *Los Angeles Times,* February 9, 1998.

11. Susan Kuner, Carol Matzkin Osborn, Linda Quigley, and Karen Leigh Stroup, *Speak the Language of Healing: Living with Breast Cancer without Going to War,* (Berkeley, CA: Conari Press, 1999), 34.

12. Susan Kuner, et al., *Speak the Language of Healing*, 52.

13. Rosie Mestel, "Need a Second Opinion?" *Los Angeles Times*, February 15, 1999, Health Section, Orange County edition.

14. Kamin, *The Path of the Soul*, 26.

15. Kubler-Ross, *On Death and Dying*, 42.

16. Mitch Albom, *Tuesdays with Morrie*, (New York: Doubleday, 1997), 83.

17. Kuner, et al., *Speak the Language of Healing*, 55–56.

18. Kamin, Cover of *The Path of the Soul*, and 8.

Lesson Five: The Medical Team

1. *The American Heritage Dictionary of the English Language*, 60.

2. Kuner, et al., *Speak the Language of Healing*, 77–78.

3. Siegel, *Love, Medicine and Miracles*, 4.

4. Landro, *Los Angeles Times*, November 2, 1998.

5. Landro, *Los Angeles Times*, November 2, 1998.

6. Marilyn Elias, "The Doctor Is Inattentive," *USA Today*, September 23, 2003, Front Section.

7. Herczog, *Los Angeles Times*, December 8, 1997.

8. Kamin, *Denial of the Soul*, 52.

9. Herczog, *Los Angeles Times*, December 8, 1997.

10. Tara Parker-Pope, "Unrestricted Visits to Hospital Rooms May Help Recovery of the Sickest Patients," *Wall Street Journal*, August 13, 2004, Health Journal.

11. Siegel, *Love, Medicine and Miracles*, 173–174.

Lesson Six: The Patient

1. Kamin, *The Path of the Soul,* 59.

2. Herczog, *Los Angeles Times,* December 8, 1997.

3. Kuner et al., *Speak the Language of Healing,* 83.

4. Kuner et al., *Speak the Language of Healing,* 26–27.

5. Matthews, *The Faith Factor,* 145.

6. Kamin, *The Path of the Soul,* 125.

7. Peck, *Denial of the Soul,* 108–109.

8. Kuner, et al., *Speak the Language of Healing,* 83.

9. Herczog, *Los Angeles Times,* February 9, 1998.

10. Herczog, *Los Angeles Times,* February 9, 1998.

11. Herczog, *Los Angeles Times,* February 9, 1998.

12. Julia Cameron, *The Artist's Way: A Spiritual Path to Higher Creativity,* (New York: Tarcher/Putnam Books, 1992), 4.

13. Herczog, *Los Angeles Times,* February 9, 1998.

Lesson Seven: The Patient's Team

1. Kamin, *The Path of the Soul,* 130.

2. Matthews, *The Faith Factor,* 250.

3. Kubler-Ross, *On Death and Dying,* 167.

Lesson Eight: Being With the Patient

1. Peck, *Denial of the Soul,* 93.

2. Kuner et al, *Speak the Language of Healing,* 41.

3. Kuner et al, *Speak the Language of Healing,* 41.

4. Remens, *Kitchen Table Wisdom*, 151.

5. Remens, *Kitchen Table Wisdom*, 244.

6. Nouwen, *Seeds of Hope*, 61.

7. Kamin, *Path of the Soul*, 144.

8. Kamin, *Path of the Soul*, 125.

9. Jean Shinoda Bolen, Introduction to *Speak the Language of Healing*, xiii.

10. Kubler-Ross, *On Death and Dying*, 151.

11. Nouwen, *Seeds of Hope*, 257.

12. Kubler-Ross, *Life Lessons*, 173.

13. Albom, *Tuesdays with Morrie*, 64–65.

14. Albom, *Tuesdays with Morrie*, 164.

15. Albom, *Tuesdays with Morrie*, 166.

16. Joel Stein, "Just Say Om," *Time Magazine*, August 4, 2003.

17. Jane Glenn Haas, "When Caregivers Give Till It Hurts," Orange County Register, December 7, 2003, Life Section.

18. Dossey, *Healing Words*, 7.

19. Dossey, Preface to *Healing Words*, xviii.

20. Schimmel, *Cancer Talk*, 286.

21. Dossey, Preface to *Healing Words*, xx.

22. Lauren Artress, PhD, *Walking a Sacred Path: Rediscovering the Labyrinth as a Spiritual Tool*, (New York: The Berkeley Group/The Penguin Group, 1992), 82.

23. Albom, *Tuesdays with Morrie*, 70.

24. Kamin, *The Path of the Soul*, 39.

25. Remens, *Kitchen Table Wisdom*, 151–153.

26. Jane Roy Brown, "Designs That Heal," Garden Design Magazine, November/December, 2004, 12.

Lesson Nine: Emotional/Psychological Support

1. Lorna Reed, Cancer Center Report, University of Southern California Norris Comprehensive Cancer Center, Winter 1999/2000.

2. Schimmel, *Cancer Talk,* p. 80.

3. Jane Glenn Haas, "Are You Overwhelmed? Here Are Some Signs," Orange County Register, December 19, 2001, Accent Section.

4. MSN Encarta Encyclopedia, Psychotherapy, http://www.encarta.msn.com/encyclopedia, accessed September 6, 2001.

5. American Academy of Psychoanalysis Web site, http://www.aapsa.org, "Frequently Asked Questions," p. 1, accessed August 20, 2001.

Lesson Ten: Self-care for Caregivers

1. Kubler-Ross, *Life Lessons,* 86.

2. Diane Rodecker, "Retreat Will Refresh Caregivers," Orange County Register, July 15, 2001, Accent Section.

3. Schimmel, *Cancer Talk,* 186.

4. Schimmel, *Cancer Talk,* 195.

5. Siegel, *Love, Medicine and Miracles,* 28.

6. Laura Claverie, "Letters," *Food and Wine Magazine,* March, 2002.

7. Ellen Rose, "Healing, Giving, Baking," *Better Homes and Gardens Magazine,* April, 2004.

8. Schimmel, *Cancer Talk,* p. 182.

9. Diane Rodecker, "Resource Center Puts the Caring First," Orange County Register, January 26, 2003, Accent Section.

10. Kubler-Ross, *Life Lessons,* 48.

Conclusion: Life Is Messy

1. Kuner, et al., *Speak the Language of Healing,* 155–156.

2. Kubler-Ross, *Life Lessons,* 23.

3. Cardinal Joseph Bernardin, *The Gift of Peace: Personal Reflections,* (New York, Image books/Doubleday, 1997), 48–49.

BIBLIOGRAPHY

Albom, Mitch, *Tuesdays with Morrie,* New York: Doubleday, 1997.

American Academy of Psychoanalysis and Dynamic Psychiatry, "Frequently Asked Questions," http://www.aapdp.org, accessed August 20, 2001.

Antenen, Jay, "The Touch That Heals," Cincinnati CityBeat, July 14–20, 2004, p. 16.

Artress, Lauren, PhD, *Walking a Sacred Path: Rediscovering the Labyrinth as a Spiritual Tool,* New York: The Berkeley Group/Penguin Group, 1992.

Bernardin, Cardinal Joseph, *The Gift of Peace: Personal Reflections,* New York: Image Books/Doubleday, 1997.

Brown, Jane Roy, "Designs That Heal," Garden Design Magazine, November/December, 2004.

Cameron, Julia, *The Artist's Way: A Spiritual Path to Higher Creativity,* New York: Tarcher/Putnam Books, 1992.

Carter, Rosalyn, with Goliant, Susan K., *Helping Yourself Help Others,* New York: Random House, 1994.

Claverie, Laura, "Letters," *Food and Wine Magazine,* March, 2002.

Cousins, Norman, *Anatomy of an Illness as Perceived by the Patient,* New York: W. W. Norton & Company, 1979.

Dossey, Larry, MD, *Healing Words: The Power of Prayer and the Practice of Medicine,* New York: Harper Paperbacks, 1993.

Durback, Robert, Ed., *Seeds of Hope: A Henri Nouwen Reader,* New York: Image Books/Doubleday, 1997.

Dyer, Wayne W., *Wisdom of the Ages: 60 Days to Enlightenment*, New York: Harper Collins, 1998.

Elias, Marilyn, "The Doctor Is Inattentive," USA Today, September 23, 2003.

Haas, Jane Glenn, "Are You Overwhelmed? Here Are Some Signs," Orange County Register, December 19, 2001, Accent Section.

Haas, Jane Glenn, "When Caregivers Give Till It Hurts," Orange County Register, December 7, 2003, Life Section.

Harrison, Charles Yale, *Thank God for My Heart Attack*, New York: Henry Holt & Co., 1949.

Herczog, Mary Susan, "A Battle with Breast Cancer," *Los Angeles Times*, December 8, 1997, Health Section, Orange County edition.

Herczog, Mary Susan, "Inside the Healing Circle," *Los Angeles Times*, February 9, 1998, Health Section, Orange County edition.

Herczog, Mary Susan, "The Who, What and Why Behind Her Treatment," *Los Angeles Times*, July, 13, 1998, Health Section, Orange County edition.

Kamin, Ben, Rabbi, *The Path of the Soul: Making Peace with Mortality*, New York: A Plume Book, 1999.

Kubler-Ross, Elisabeth, MD, and Kessler, David, *Life Lessons*, New York: Scribner, 2000.

Kubler-Ross, Elisabeth, MD, *On Death and Dying*, New York: Touchstone Books/Simon & Schuster, 1969.

Kuner, Susan; Orsborn, Carol Matzkin; Quigley, Linda, and Stroup, Karen Leigh, *Speak the Language of Healing: Living with Breast Cancer without Going to War*, Berkeley, CA: Conari Press, 1999.

Landro, Laura, "Be Your Own Greatest Ally in Battling Cancer," *Los Angeles Times,* November 2, 1998, Health Section, Orange County edition.

Matthews, Dale, MD, with Clark, Connie, *The Faith Factor: Proof of the Healing Power of Prayer,* New York: Penguin Books, 1998.

Mestel, Rosie, "Need A Second Opinion?" *Los Angeles Times,* February 15, 1999, Health Section, Orange County edition.

Morris, William, Ed., *The American Heritage Dictionary of the English Language, New College Edition,* Boston: Houghton Mifflin, 1979.

MSN Encarta Encyclopedia, "Psychotherapy," http://www.encarta.msn.com/encyclopedia, accessed September 6, 2001.

Osbon, Diane K., Ed., *A Joseph Campbell Companion: Reflections of the Art of Living,* New York: Harper Collins, 1991.

Palmer R.R. and Colton, Joel, *A History of the Modern World,* New York: Alfred A. Knopf, 1965.

Parker-Pope, Tara, "Unrestricted Visits to Hospital Rooms May Help Recovery of the Sickest Patients," *Wall Street Journal,* August 13, 2004, Health Journal.

Peck, M. Scott, MD, *Denial of the Soul: Spiritual and Medical Perspectives on Euthanasia and Mortality,* New York: Harmony Books, 1997.

Reed, Lorna, Cancer Center Report, University of Southern California Norris Comprehensive Cancer Center, Winter 1999/2000.

Remens, Rachel Naomi, MD, *Kitchen Table Wisdom: Stories That Heal,* New York: Riverhead Books, 1996.

Rodecker, Diane, "Retreat Will Refresh Caregivers," Orange County Register, July 15, 2001, Accent Section.

Rodecker, Diane, "Resource Center Puts the Caring First," Orange County Register, January 26, 2003, Accent Section.

Rose, Ellen, "Healing, Giving, Baking," *Better Homes and Gardens Magazine,* April, 2004.

Schimmel, Selma R., with Barry Fox, PhD, *Cancer Talk,* New York: Broadway Books, 1999.

Schulz, Richard, PhD, and Beach, Scott R., PhD, Abstract, "Caregiving as a Risk Factor for Mortality: The Caregiver Health Effects Study," *Journal of the American Medical Association,* December, 1999.

Siegel, Bernie S., MD, *Love, Medicine and Miracles,* New York: Harper Perennial, 1986.

Siegel, Bernie S., MD, *Peace, Love and Healing,* New York: Harper Perennial, 1989.

The Inner Treasure: An Introduction to the World's Scared and Mystical Writings, Starr, Jonathan, ed., New York: Tarcher/Putnam, 1999.

Stein, Joel, "Just Say Om," *Time Magazine,* August 4, 2003.

Weil, Andrew, MD, *Sound Body, Sound Mind: Music for Healing,* CD and book, Los Angeles: Rhino Recordings/Wea, 2005.